ADVANCE PRAISE FOR
IDENTITY THEFT: REDISCOVERING OURSELVES AFTER STROKE

"After watching Debra Meyerson's extraordinary academic career cut short by her debilitating stroke, it is so inspiring to see her create such a powerful book for anyone trying to build a life of meaning in the face of adversity."

—CLAUDE STEELE, PROFESSOR EMERITUS OF PSYCHOLOGY, STANFORD UNIVERSITY, AND FORMER DEAN, STANFORD SCHOOL OF EDUCATION; AUTHOR OF *WHISTLING VIVALDI*

• • •

"*Identity Theft* is a scholarly yet easy-to-read exposition that addresses so many issues faced by stroke survivors, especially those with aphasia. It is a story of determination and hope that should be of interest to everyone."

—LEORA R. CHERNEY, PHD, SCIENTIFIC CHAIR, THINK + SPEAK LAB, SHIRLEY RYAN ABILITYLAB; PROFESSOR, PHYSICAL MEDICINE & REHABILITATION, NORTHWESTERN UNIVERSITY

• • •

"It is a rare book that can begin with medical trauma and loss of self-identity and turn into a deeply moving, surprisingly uplifting, and profoundly wise meditation on what it means to be human."

—ROB REICH, PROFESSOR OF POLITICAL SCIENCE, STANFORD UNIVERSITY; AUTHOR OF *JUST GIVING*

• • •

"With *Identity Theft*, Debra Meyerson has written what will certainly become a go-to resource for stroke survivors and their families, navigating that critical question—'Who do I want to be now?'"

—JULIA FOX GARRISON, STROKE SURVIVOR AND MOTIVATIONAL SPEAKER, BESTSELLING AUTHOR OF *DON'T LEAVE ME THIS WAY*

• • •

"*Identity Theft* offers a deeply moving, candid, eye-opening, and compassionate picture of life after stroke. It displays the power of resilience, determination, acceptance, and love—and is sure to inspire helpful reflection, no matter one's age or health."

—KATHERINE J. KLEIN, EDWARD H. BOWMAN PROFESSOR OF MANAGEMENT AND VICE DEAN, WHARTON SOCIAL IMPACT INITIATIVE, THE WHARTON SCHOOL, UNIVERSITY OF PENNSYLVANIA

OTHER BOOKS BY DEBRA E. MEYERSON

Tempered Radicals:
How People Use Difference to Inspire Change at Work
(reprinted as: Rocking the Boat: How Tempered Radicals
Effect Change Without Making Trouble)

Preparing Principals for a Changing World
Lessons From Effective School Leadership Programs

Identity Theft

REDISCOVERING OURSELVES AFTER STROKE

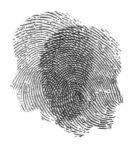

DEBRA E. MEYERSON, PhD
WITH **DANNY ZUCKERMAN**

SPECIAL THANKS TO SALLY COLLINGS, CONTRIBUTOR

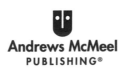

Andrews McMeel
PUBLISHING®

DEDICATION

To Steve—my husband, partner, lover, playmate,
best friend, and unnamed coauthor—
you are a truly incredible supporter in stroke recovery and life.

Contents

Introduction

"**M**y name is Debra Meyerson." In 2009, this was a casual self-introduction at the beginning of a lecture at Stanford University. The tone was strong and authoritative, five words opening the door to thousands more over the course of two hours as I confidently led a class through a presentation and discussion about topics like gender, diversity, social change, and identity.

"My name is Debra Meyerson." In 2011, this same phrase comes out weak, a faltering melody with an almost nursery-rhyme cadence. The five uneven words are an achievement, the result of a year of speech therapy. A severe stroke in September 2010 robbed me of all speech, and after a year of intensive therapy, my own name still gave me trouble. In times of stress or fatigue, I still fall back on singing the phrase, using a melody to unlock the words.

"My name is Debra Meyerson." Who is Debra Meyerson now, in 2018, as I write this book? I am alive, and for that I am lucky and grateful. I live with significant disabilities: no functional use of my right hand, a significant limp, and significantly diminished speech. I can say my own name, and much more, but at times I still struggle to find the simplest of words. This brings me to laughter on my good days and tears of frustration on the bad. I cherish the same values, love the same family, work with the same determination. But I can no longer teach, talk as easily with family and friends, or ride a bike on my own.

"My name is Debra Meyerson." Strokes don't just create physical and mental disabilities, they can also steal our identities. Much of my pre-stroke life became inaccessible. Understanding and accepting the loss of my old life

1

was one of the hardest parts of my recovery and rebuilding process. Along with the constant rehab and speech therapy aimed at physical recovery, I've spent the past eight years working to regain my sense of self, trying to answer the question: who am I now?

. . .

As a professor at Stanford's Graduate School of Education and Graduate School of Business for fifteen years, I studied how personal identity shapes people's experiences in their organizational lives. My first book, *Tempered Radicals: How People Use Difference to Inspire Change at Work* (since reprinted as *Rocking the Boat: How Tempered Radicals Effect Change Without Making Trouble*),[1] examined people who maintained multiple identities and worked to align their personal and organizational lives. I had planned to continue this work, building and sharing knowledge about how each of our identities shapes our experiences and our environments. Had I been able to proceed with that work, perhaps I would now be publishing a book exploring how we can use a more complete understanding of our multiple identities to improve the way organizations handle difference and conflict.

Instead, I find myself grappling to understand my own identity. My stroke took away my capacity to work as I did before, many of my abilities, and many of the other pieces of the life I had built over five decades. Although my physical capabilities were erased nearly overnight, there was no analogous "identity switch" that signaled how my sense of self had changed. But over time, this change became clear. Activities I loved were out of reach; colleagues, friends, and strangers treated me differently; family dynamics changed dramatically. I even noticed my own attitude changing in certain ways.

I have gradually regained some of the capabilities I initially lost, and the recovery of my identity has been an equally difficult journey, one that took me about three years to even recognize. Following my stroke, I found numerous resources to help me understand my journey to recover physically, but there was a profound lack of guidance when I faced the emotional challenge of rebuilding my sense of self in this new and maddening circumstance. As I talked with other stroke survivors, I found this to be an extremely common frustration.

For many of us, clarifying essential elements of our selves is critical to regaining capability and confidence, whatever physical challenges remain. As we try to restore parts of the identities we had before the stroke, we are also reinventing new ones—all the while grasping for tools to help us think about how our lives should be evolving. Do we stay determined not to let the stroke win and keep battling for more recovery? Or do we accept that we need to let go of our past selves? Or both?

I was confused and struggling. But I was still thinking like a social scientist. I tried to make sense of the experiences that I and others in my new community of survivors were going through. Was their sense of self shattered like mine? How did it evolve with time? Did they ever lose hope? How did they balance the time and rigor of rehabilitation with an acceptance of their newfound limitations? How did they maximize life within those constraints? Did they, as I did, eventually discover some silver linings—ways in which some things were actually better after stroke, in spite of all the frustrations?

While exploring these questions, I was ushered into a whole community built around poststroke life—a community I never had reason to notice before. I encountered it at therapy centers and speech clinics, through survivor support groups meeting in coffee shops, on Facebook and other online groups. I actually started to notice similar dynamics in other communities, as well—colleagues struggling with the loss of a partner, survivors recovering from brain injuries, and even just friends facing the realities of older age. The more I thought and talked about it, the more I realized how many of us are united in this journey to understand and shape our own identities in the face of life changes.

In the stroke community, whenever talk turned to the question of self-image and the psychological impact of stroke, people's eyes lit up with interest. Yet, I met very few survivors who had received any kind of formal psychological support or counseling; at best, some had benefited from talking with an empathetic speech or physical therapist. This is hardly surprising, given that many survivors receive only the barest of physical and occupational therapy, let alone emotional counseling.

I realized that telling the story of my own journey might assist other survivors, as well as those who love and support them. And, frankly, I knew the process would help me better understand my own experience and allow me to reclaim what I loved most about being a professor: helping to create and share knowledge. I also knew I wanted to share the stories of other stroke survivors. As I talked with them, I discovered many similarities, but I found the equally numerous differences in our experiences even more interesting. Their stories became part of mine, expanding my understanding and shaping this book with a broader perspective that I hope will be more helpful to the survivor community than just my own.

Every person is different. Every stroke is different. Every recovery is different. Mark Wells had a major stroke three days after his son was murdered. Andrea Helft, a former business consultant, was stripped of her ability to remember even the simplest conversation. Rocio Rojas was just thirty-two when she suffered a stroke two weeks after giving birth to her first child. Mary Jones's husband filed for divorce and shipped her off to relatives when her care became too arduous. Emmanuel "Manny" Gigante was a hard-driving, money-driven young man whose stroke slowed him down and showed him the rewards to be found in helping others.

These are just a handful of the incredible people I got to know while writing this book. In the pages that follow, I'll share small pieces of the incredible journeys of several dozen stroke survivors and many of their family members and caregivers. The survivors are men and women of all races and backgrounds; wealthy, comfortable, and of very modest means; as young as thirteen and as old as sixty-five at the time of their strokes; living in cities and towns throughout the United States. Some I have identified by their real names; others asked that I use a pseudonym.

Many of these survivors have found friendship, solace, and meaning in the stroke community. Most of the people I have spoken with have been remarkably optimistic and positive given the circumstances. A few, like Andrea Helft, have even suggested that in some ways they are happier now. Others, like Malik Thoma, have had a more difficult time grappling with the aftermath. A few I spoke with are struggling with severe depression—one has even attempted suicide.

Their stories expose some of the highest and lowest points of human experience, both for the stroke survivors and for the families and caretakers around them. Our individual journeys were influenced not just by the nature, severity, and duration of our disabilities but also by background, gender, income level, race, ethnicity, profession, outlook, age, and many other factors that shape identity. Because of this, we each struggle with different aspects of this journey, and the entire experience is harder for some than for others. This is not fair, but it is reality. And the one thing we all do have in common is that we now own "stroke survivor" as a facet of our identity as we try to navigate who we are and who we will become.

As I worked on this book, I talked with friends and colleagues who assured me that the issues I was wrestling with were equally present for people who had experienced traumatic brain injuries and other catastrophic health issues, as well as their supporters. In fact, many healthy friends found this journey relevant as they struggled with their concept of self while growing older, retiring, getting divorced, or navigating other major life transitions. All of these circumstances can prompt the kind of reflection and self-examination that reaches deep beneath the surface of jobs and family roles, chores and hobbies. A traumatic event like stroke seems to shine a spotlight on broader issues of identity, regardless of health.

I do not claim to have "figured it out." Quite the contrary. Despite my expertise in identity and all the time I have spent thinking about it with respect to recovering from my stroke, I still grapple with my own identity on a near daily basis. A vital part of my rebuilding process has been acknowledging, and sometimes even celebrating, my identity as a stroke survivor. That did not come quickly or easily. In the first months, I resisted letting people know that I had even had a stroke. I viewed it as a temporary status, a superficial condition that interrupted the normal life I would return to soon. Today, it is one of the first things I share when meeting new people. I am no longer able to be a tenured professor. By embracing my stroke as part of my identity—and writing this book—I can explore and generate knowledge and teach in a new way. Instead of trying to re-create a lesser version of my prior self, I am working to integrate my new identity as a survivor with my old one as an educator, and in doing so I can do things I simply couldn't do before.

Don't get me wrong: having a stroke *sucks.* For me, it sucks in all the everyday tasks that used to be so easy but which are now time-consuming struggles. It sucks every time I miss out on a conversation I would love to be a part of because the words just won't come out fast enough. It sucks for my husband Steve, who has to do so much more to help me—from little things like putting in my contact lenses to big things like taking lots of time away from a job he loves to help me so much with this book. It sucks that we probably won't be able to retire onto a boat as we grow old together, something we had long envisioned. It sucks for our kids, who can't interact and talk with their mom in the same ways they did before; they also feel an added responsibility to stay close and be there to support me, just as they are beginning to build their own adult lives. It sucks for all the friends and colleagues I've known for years, and simply can't keep up with given my lessened abilities.

Remarkably though, there really are some things that are better since my stroke, and it's been crucial for me to acknowledge and talk about them. I laugh more, and more deeply. I appreciate food like never before. I've had (or made) more time in my life for friends and have developed some incredible new relationships. There are ways in which I feel even closer to my family, and we were very close before. Creating space to celebrate these and other positives certainly doesn't mean I'm glad I had a stroke, but it has been immensely helpful in my efforts to move forward.

The life I have made for myself since my stroke is a good and full life. It is not at all the life I used to have, nor is it the life I once imagined for myself. I am acutely aware that I'm privileged to have what I have, even though there are times when I feel depressed, frustrated, and angry. Some of the people featured in this book have found a more positive balance than I have, while others have experienced a more difficult road. We are all at a different place in our journeys, and all have different lessons to share. The people whose stories make up the pages that follow have gone over the mountains and into the valleys of recovery. This book exists because I wanted to share our stories, and some of what we have learned, in a way that might help other survivors accelerate their poststroke journeys to recover, rediscover themselves, and rebuild a fulfilling life.

• • •

As it turns out, wanting and doing are two very different things. Eight years after my stroke, I still live in a world where a brief conversation can leave me noticeably fatigued, and a three-sentence email can take twenty minutes to write. For almost three years, my full-time job was to relearn some fundamental skills I had lost—how to walk, raise my right arm, and say a sentence clearly. That kind of therapy continues to fill a good bit of my life today and will likely continue to do so for the foreseeable future.

I have returned to the classroom on a few occasions and have delivered brief presentations to a few understanding groups. But professionally, I am certainly not back to where I was before.

When I first started contemplating this book, it was still difficult for me to clearly articulate even a simple question like, "When did your stroke occur?" More interesting questions, like, "How has your relationship with your spouse and kids changed since your stroke?" were impossible. And note-taking: not a chance. Clearly, I was going to need some help to tell this story. Just as tandem bike riding had replaced solo cycling for me, what once would have been an individual effort would clearly require teamwork.

For three years, writer and editor Sally Collings was my partner. She put words to my ideas, did the bulk of the talking in our dozens of interviews, and extracted my story through hours of conversation. She did research on identity and trauma and combed through my own academic history to better understand my perspectives. She offered ideas I might include in the book, and I would then confirm or point her in different directions. She, Steve, and I talked about structure, reviewed and refined her chapter outlines and early drafts. Sally wove all of this into a complete first draft of this book.

That draft didn't quite capture the full message I wanted to deliver, so with her contract complete, the book became a family effort. My oldest son Danny, then between jobs, took up the pen and became the principal drafter. With help from Steve and our two other kids—Adam and Sarah— we restructured the book, refined the message, revised Sally's content, and redrafted (and redrafted, and redrafted) into this final version.

This book is written in three parts. Part One is largely my journey through the world of stroke, recovery, and shifting identity. Woven throughout are stories of other survivors. Many of their stories are shared more fully in Part Two, where each chapter is dedicated to exploring a particularly critical challenge in the physical and emotional aftermath of strokes. Part Three concludes with a summary of the lessons we've collectively learned about rebuilding an identity and a fulfilling life through this journey.

We have written this book in the first person singular because it is, in large part, my story. However, in many places, "I" reflects the "we" of my writing partnership with Danny, Sally, Steve, Adam, and Sarah, who were all a critical part of the writing team. This collaboration is a good example of how life has changed for me, and most of us, after stroke.

PART ONE:

UNWINDING
a Self

CHAPTER 1.

A Slow Fall off a Cliff

It was Labor Day weekend 2010. I had just dropped off our middle child, Adam, in Boston to start college at Tufts University. Shaking off the bittersweet emotions, I was heading to Lake Tahoe for a relaxing pre-school weekend with the rest of my family—my husband Steve, our oldest son Danny, and our youngest, Sarah. On the drive early Saturday morning, I told Steve, "My right leg feels weird."

I had no more precise word for the feeling. It was neither uncomfortable nor painful, not numb or asleep, just . . . not right. I figured a good walk would help shake it out, so when we arrived four hours later, we set out for our favorite hike up Shirley Canyon behind the Squaw Valley ski area. I could walk without problem, but this hike involved some scrambles and bouldering, and my leg would buckle when I bent it beyond forty-five degrees. It felt weak, and I couldn't step up or down as I normally could. The kids went on with our dog Kaya, but Steve and I turned around and went back to the condo. I had a bit of a headache, so I took some aspirin. Over dinner, we speculated about pinched nerves, misalignments, and inactive muscles.

On Sunday morning, my headache was worse. When Steve held out the aspirin I had asked him for, he watched my right arm move very slowly toward the two pills in his palm. He noticed that I had to concentrate with all my strength to compel my fingers to pick up the pills. I actually didn't notice anything strange. Steve did. Right leg, right arm, headache. "We're going to the hospital," he told me. It seemed ridiculous to be making such

12

a fuss, and I tried to convince him that we should just drive home and deal with it there. Thankfully, he didn't listen to me.

At Tahoe Forest Hospital in nearby Truckee, Steve and Danny watched me fail several physical tests as a doctor asked me to identify which toe he was touching and to move my right arm in specific ways. They quickly moved me to the imaging lab and a CT scan confirmed their expectations. They told us I'd had an "ischemic event." They put me in an ambulance to Renown Hospital, thirty-four miles away in Reno, where they have a full neurology practice and stroke unit. Steve rode with me, trying to keep calm as we sat in painfully slow traffic that eventually forced the ambulance to move into the shoulder. Danny trailed us in our car also trying to keep calm while he phoned his premed college friends to find out what the hell an "ischemic event" meant. Should he be panicking? He called Sarah, who had stayed at the condo with our dog Kaya, to give her a vague update and ask her to hang tight.

Two hours after arrival at Renown Hospital, I had been through an MRI, and the diagnosis was confirmed as a stroke. Sitting in the emergency room that afternoon, I seemed relatively stable. I talked on the phone to both Adam and my brother, Aaron. I told them I was concerned I might miss the start of the fall class I was supposed to teach at Stanford in a couple of weeks. Steve said my speech in those conversations was beginning to slur, but I didn't notice. The doctors weren't telling us much about what to expect, and they were completely noncommittal about how things might progress. They hinted at a few treatments they had in mind but weren't ready to go ahead with yet.

Without much information from the doctors, my family had to figure out how to react. Danny, about to start his senior year of college, began hearing back from his friends. "I was hoping someone was going to tell me, 'Oh, it's fine. You're freaking out over something that's probably nothing.' But instead, I was hearing, 'Take it seriously.'" When Adam got the call from Steve on Monday afternoon to say that I'd had a stroke, he had no idea whether that might simply mean an overnight stay in the hospital or the loss of his mom forever. This is serious, Steve told him, "We'd love for you to come home." Steve is not prone to panic, so even before he started his web search, Adam knew it was really serious. The next day, he caught an early morning flight from Boston. Sarah, then a high school sophomore, admits she was completely ignorant, as most of us are until stroke hits close to home. "I didn't know how bad strokes could be, because I'd never come face-to-face with one. I was imagining the worst, but I also had no idea what to expect. I didn't know what 'she's having a stroke' could possibly mean."

The medical team was clear on the stroke diagnosis, but they still had very little clarity about the cause. When they finally moved me to a room on the stroke floor at about 10 p.m., I was frustrated. At least, I'm told I was—I don't remember much from these days. Danny and Steve do, and they were getting more scared. I didn't know it at the time, but my condition was getting much worse.

. . .

A stroke is the sudden death of brain cells in a localized area caused by insufficient oxygen to a part of the brain. In more technical circles, it is called a cerebrovascular insult—a term that seems particularly fitting to those who survive it. Sometimes it's simply called a brain attack. About 85 percent of strokes are ischemic strokes, which occur when an artery bringing blood to the brain becomes narrowed or blocked, causing severely reduced blood flow (ischemia) and the death of brain cells. Most ischemic strokes are caused by a buildup of plaque inside an artery and/or a blood clot lodging itself in an artery. Other strokes are called hemorrhagic strokes, caused by a rupture or leak in a blood vessel in the brain that floods brain cells with too much blood, effectively drowning brain cells to death.

Quickly recognizing a stroke and its cause is critical. In promoting stroke awareness and the importance of a rapid response, Pacific Stroke Association, like many others, uses the acronym FAST. Posters explain:

FACE - Look for an uneven smile.
ARM - Check if one arm is weak.
SPEECH - Listen for slurred speech.
TIME - Call 911 right away.

Time is critical after a stroke because there are now treatments that can dramatically reduce the damage caused by a stroke if applied quickly. Most notable is tissue plasminogen activator (tPA), sometimes called the clot buster. If a blood clot is causing the stroke, administration of tPA within four hours can break up the clot and restore blood flow to the brain, eliminating or significantly reducing the amount of permanent damage. This treatment has been incredibly successful. It's tricky, though. In a hemorrhagic stroke, tPA would amplify the bleeding and could cause death. There are also new minimally invasive surgical procedures in which a doctor can thread a device into your arteries, find a clot and physically remove it.

Unknown to any of us at the time, in my case the blood being pumped from my heart up to the left side of my brain had run into a traffic jam. Much later, we learned that my cerebral carotid artery had developed a small tear in the innermost layer of its multilayered structure—something called a dissection. It's not a common problem, and in most of the limited cases when it happens, blood flow pushes the resulting flap of tissue back against the wall, and it repairs itself without any ill effects. However, in my case, blood had begun to accumulate between the layers, effectively narrowing the artery and preventing some of the normal blood flow from getting to the left side of my brain. At some point, the blood flow was stopped completely. I was still getting some collateral blood flow from the carotid artery on my right side, but not nearly enough. An area of my brain called the watershed wasn't getting sufficient blood, and brain cells were dying.

We had no idea about any of this at the time, and neither did the doctors. I just had a weird feeling in my leg and a relatively mild headache, then some trouble walking, then reaching, and then speaking. One of the emotionally difficult characteristics of stroke is that it often comes swiftly and with no apparent prompt or cause.[2] It also can take some time for the full extent of the damage to reveal itself even after the event is over.

• • •

Between Sunday evening and Monday morning, the impact of my stroke was becoming more apparent and more extreme. At 10 p.m., when I had been moved onto the Neurology floor, my speech was awkward but still clear. I had started to exhibit confusion and had more obvious problems moving my right leg and arm. After the 11 p.m. shift change, a nurse told Steve that it often takes awhile for the full damage of the stroke to reveal itself, and that arms usually lose function faster and more completely than legs. She said that the MRI taken Sunday night showed no additional damage compared to the one taken when I arrived, but he shouldn't be surprised to see more physical deterioration.

They woke me every hour through the night to do a standard neurological exam, asking me to move my arms and legs and try to describe pictures on a page. Every hour, I was a bit worse. "I felt completely helpless," Steve remembered. "Deb was clearly getting worse, but they kept telling me there's nothing they can do to affect the path of her decline. I kept thinking there had to be something they could do . . . something I could do. And there just wasn't. I had no idea what the bottom of the slide would be. Death? A coma? Complete paralysis?"

We've come to describe that night as my slow-motion fall off a cliff. By morning, my right side was almost completely paralyzed. My arm was immobile, and I could just barely twitch my leg. The right side of my face had "stroke droop." With each hourly exam, my speech had become more slurred, then soft, then stunted. At the 8:00 a.m. exam, I was completely mute. I couldn't even pass a cough through my lips.

Steve said he could tell I was "still there" when he looked into my eyes. But I couldn't have told him he was right, because I had lost the ability to form words, or even sounds. I don't know if I could hear and comprehend what he was saying to me, since I have no recollection of those first few days.

Steve and Danny thought I was getting good care in Renown Hospital, but it had become clear that I was not going to bounce back from this quickly. We were learning that a stroke as severe as mine could easily require a week or more in the hospital and lots of therapy after that. Steve decided it would be best to get me down to Stanford Hospital as soon as possible. Not only does Stanford have a world-class stroke center, but it is also just ten minutes from our home and close to our strongest support network of friends. He wanted to set up near home for whatever lay ahead. The doctors said that, medically, I was stable enough for a transfer. We got lucky with logistics, and a transfer for Steve and me was arranged for late that night.

Danny, Sarah and Kaya drove back to the Bay Area. My mom arranged a flight from her home in Los Angeles and actually beat us to Stanford Hospital. Adam was en route from Boston. I arrived there just after midnight on September 7, 2010, and was taken straight to the intensive care unit (ICU).

Most stroke survivors remain in the hospital, usually in a stroke unit, for up to week to ensure they are medically stable and ready for more intensive therapy. The goal is usually to get the survivor into an inpatient therapy center as quickly as possible because rehab is more effective the sooner it starts after stroke. Unfortunately, the cause of my stroke baffled the doctors. I was experiencing medical complications, and I therefore required close supervision and a lot of testing.

For two weeks, my family watched my condition hover in Stanford's ICU. I still had no speech, virtually no movement on my right side, no feeling in my right arm, and that right-side face droop. The swallowing reflex on my right side wasn't functioning properly, so a speech therapist had me practice chewing and swallowing ice. Until I gained more control over my throat and got past the risk of choking on my food, I was nourished through a feeding tube inserted in my nose. I could barely force an occasional lopsided smile— not out of pleasure but to reassure my family I was still there.

It wasn't the severity of my symptoms that kept me in the ICU. Because the doctors still didn't know the cause of my dissection, they couldn't effectively evaluate the potential risks that small changes in my blood pressure and other medical symptoms could pose. The more careful monitoring provided in the ICU was essential. My family stayed on edge. They were starving for information, but there were no clear answers. My husband Steve provided regular updates for friends and family on Caringbridge.org, a great website that makes it easy to share updates and receive support. On September 18, after eleven days in the ICU, he wrote:

> *What has been most confusing is Deb's current medical condition, and the efforts to understand the cause of the initial stroke. It truly is a reality check that medicine—at least regarding strokes— is as much art as science. And that as much as we talk about the "images" that the doctors review . . . they only give the radiologists and doctors representative data from which to draw inferences. Bottom line—they KNOW very little from these pictures, they just get data around which they can form hypotheses.*

So, while doctors tried to make sense of the data, my family tried to make sense of what they saw: their mom, wife, daughter, sister lying mute and mostly immobile in the ICU. "I don't know that I fully understood it until I saw her in the hospital, not able to talk or move," my mom recalled later. "I don't know Deb as helpless, and it was devastating. It was terrifying and depressing and horrible, the whole ball of wax."

My family watched as teams of doctors from the stroke center rotated through the ICU to evaluate my condition. Some days a little better, some days worse. Lots of theories and updates, but seemingly no answers. My stroke was not typical. Then again, no stroke is.

· · ·

About eight hundred thousand people experience a stroke each year in the United States. Strokes afflict young and old, rich and poor, urban and rural, active and sedentary.[3] A quarter of strokes occur in people younger than sixty-five years of age. Plenty of us had few or no traditional risk factors or family history.

The World Health Organization has defined stroke as a "neurological deficit of cerebrovascular cause that persists beyond twenty-four hours or is interrupted by death within twenty-four hours."[4] Thanks to declining stroke mortality, people are increasingly likely to live with the aftermath of stroke rather than dying from it. All of the people in this book are among the lucky ones in at least one way: our strokes were not interrupted by death.

With brain damage, a millimeter to the left, right, up, or down, can make the difference between minor impairment, severe disability, or death. The symptoms of stroke are so diverse they can easily lead to misdiagnosis. A number of the stroke survivors I spoke with told me that they were diagnosed with migraine headaches or dehydration. The medical staff thought one woman who experienced visual disturbances was taking drugs or alcohol.[5] It can be difficult to get the diagnosis right away.

All of our strokes were different, so we each were, and in most cases still are, battling through a different combination of challenges: paralysis, weakness, balance problems, seizures, loss of speech, diminished expression and/or comprehension, blurry or lost vision, fatigue, memory deficits, depression, apathy, mania, and more. Just as our symptoms are different, so have been our recoveries, reactions, and even our experiences of the stroke event itself.

Thirteen-year-old Isaiah Custodio was at football practice when a crushing headache stopped him mid-stride. He jogged over to the fence intending to sit down, but before he got there, he fell to the ground and vomited. "Someone asked me what was wrong, and all I could say was, 'Help. Home. Hurt,'" Isaiah recalled. "They put me in the car, and I fainted. I saw two angels, right then and there."

Kathy Howard was celebrating her thirty-first wedding anniversary and felt a nagging indigestion (a symptom she now knows can be an early sign of stroke or heart attack for women).[6] As she went to sit on the couch after dinner, "It was almost like a zipper was installed here," she pointed to her back, "and I just felt this *wjjjjjt* right to the top of my head. When I looked at the TV, there was a big black hole in the screen. Then I got sick, and I saw red and green." Kathy and her husband Jim drove to the hospital, not sure what was wrong but pretty sure it was serious. She had suffered a severe ischemic stroke; a blood vessel had become blocked.

Sean Maloney was once considered by many to be the "anointed one"—in line to be tech giant Intel's next CEO. Sean remembers his stroke as fairly peaceful. He explained, "I said to my son, 'I really feel weird.' Bam! My carotid artery shut. I felt peaceful lying down. I looked up at the skies, and I thought, 'That's it. I'm gone.'"

Jill Bolte Taylor, a Harvard-trained brain scientist, told her stroke story in her book, *My Stroke of Insight*. She tells in great detail the feelings she had when a massive hemorrhage attacked her brain, feeling detached from herself, viewing what was happening from a distance. She observed her loss of fluid movement, realized she was having a stroke, orchestrated her own rescue (she was at home alone) with a marginally intelligible phone call, and remembers wondering how bad the damage would be if she lived and whether she could recover.[7]

Cindy Lopez, a Massachusetts-based grant manager, remembers much of her stroke but was very unaware of the severity at the time. "Even when I went to the hospital, it was so odd because, in my mind, I was OK," she recalled. She scolded her husband for telling the ambulance team she was having a stroke, thinking she was fine. "It wasn't until two days later that I realized I couldn't actually move parts of my body."

. . .

I can't say exactly when I regained some awareness of my situation. But nothing could have prepared me for what I began to understand about my condition. I was largely immobile, completely dependent, and I couldn't scream, shout, ask questions, or describe what I was feeling. I was mute. I couldn't even nod yes or shake my head no to answer a simple question.

I hadn't just lost control; I seemed to be constantly losing more of it. A week after my initial stroke, the strength I had in my right leg seemed to vanish. An MRI showed that there were no new infarcts (stroke incidents), but areas of initially healthy brain tissue around the original stroke site continued to die. We still weren't sure what had caused my stroke. Doctors could see that the main artery carrying blood to the left side of my brain had developed a tear in its inner lining, but without knowing why it had happened, they couldn't assess the likelihood of another tear. So, there were still no clear answers. As I was finally being transferred to a rehab facility, Steve wrote in CaringBridge:

> *The Docs at Stanford still haven't figured out what caused Deb's*
> *original occlusion in the left carotid artery. In something of an*
> *exit conference when we left the ICU, one of them said that if*

*he were a betting man, he'd go 60% dissection, 40% clot. To
which Aaron (Deb's brother) said with his characteristic candor,
"That's not much different from 50/50—you haven't got a clue."
The good news, as I think I've said before, is that the treatment
protocol is the same. They can't find any indication of specific risk
factors for more clotting, and the artery IS flowing—that's what
really matters. It's frustrating for my logical mind not to have
an explanation, but to paraphrase Yoda from Star Wars—"Live
with it, I will."*

The uncertainty and lack of control was excruciating. When I heard
the doctors conferring with Steve and my mom in the hall, I would lose my
temper. I wanted to be included. Even though I couldn't grasp what was
happening to me, if I had to have a medical team and a treatment program,
then I wanted to be a part of it. I felt betrayed by my body, and now I didn't
even have a say in trying to fix it. Emotions, which I don't remember having
the first days after the stroke, had definitely started to build. I felt confused.
I felt helpless. I felt broken.

During these uncertain first two months of my recovery, I found myself
grasping for connections to the outside world. Proof that not everything
had changed. My brother Aaron came for visiting hours with his iPad to
show me a slideshow of his recent family vacation. Stuck in the bubble of
the ICU, it was somehow a relief to see that life continued outside those
four walls. Aaron told me about a bike ride they took along a river. It was
supposed to be five miles and turned out to be twenty. My teenage niece,
Izzy, was so pissed off at him, she threatened to fling herself into the river.
I let out a sound—not quite a laugh but close to it. I was beaming inside at
this new sound, and looking at the faces around me, I knew the others saw
the importance of such a small development, too. A competition started
in the hospital room to see if others could find things to make me laugh.

Adam started telling me about his first weeks at Tufts, where he planned to study political science. "I need to figure out how to fulfill my fine arts requirement," he mused. "I'm thinking of taking Introduction to Salsa Dancing." Again, I made a gurgling almost-laugh.

Inevitably, though, visiting hours would end and I was left alone with my fears, with no ability to voice them. Lying in the ICU at Stanford Hospital, a frequent thought for me was that life without speech would be no better than life in a cell. I couldn't imagine being cut off from the people I love, unable to communicate with them. To accept this reality was unthinkable, but for now it was my reality.

CHAPTER 2.

Everything Can Fail

In late September, three weeks after my stroke, Danny came to visit me in my fourth hospital, Santa Clara Valley Medical Center. I was in their inpatient Acute Rehabilitation Program, a common second step for survivors of moderate to severe strokes. Steve had just gone back to work, a much-needed return to some normalcy for him, and Danny was driving down to attend my first speech-therapy session. Before departing Stanford, I had regained the ability to make some noise, but still no speech.

Jonathan was the young speech therapist assigned to me. He was cheerful and inquisitive. He started by asking me some questions, gauging my capabilities and my attitude. He saw how desperately I wanted to reply when he asked my name, how every working gear in my mind was cranking to get the words out. He saw how scared I was as I couldn't muster a coherent sound. I was terrified, but Jonathan wasn't deterred.

"No problem, let's start simple." He began to sing "Happy Birthday" and asked me to hum along. He moved his arms as he went and swung my arms with his, getting me in sync. My head started to move along with the rhythm. I started to hum along roughly in time with the music, though very out of tune. He got to the end and told me to watch his lips carefully and follow along. Then he started singing again. Danny captured the scene in CaringBridge that night:

On the second time through, on the last verse, Jonathan finished "Happy Birthday to—," and though he closed his lips on the last word, there was a clear, loud, and distinctly female "You" to the close! I didn't quite believe it at first, but looking at the shock on my mom's face, it was obvious she had just blurted out her first clear word.

I expected him to reinforce the breakthrough that had just occurred, and my mom clearly wanted to keep at the happy birthday singalong, but Jonathan immediately moved on to "Row, Row, Row Your Boat." Again, the second time through Jonathan quieted his voice, this time for the entire last verse. Mom gave a slightly garbled "Merrily, Merrily, Merrily," but the real shock came when she finished, with nearly as clear and strong a voice as normal, "Life is but a dream!" I was smiling more than I can ever remember, but it was nothing compared to the look of pure delight and surprise on my mom's face. She was crying with happiness and excitement as they started singing again, and she continued to get stronger, at times voicing every word in the nursery rhyme.

Jonathan paused to explain that, although speech is controlled by the (now damaged) left side of my brain, rhythm and melody is controlled by the right side of the brain, which was not affected by my stroke. He was using familiar songs to unlock my fluency and allow me to produce some words. Next, he created a tune for me to sing, "My name is Debra Meyerson." He started chanting it over and over, swinging my arms to it. On the third try, my voice joined his, "My name is Debra Meyerson," I sang, and my eyes teared up again. I chanted over and over, "My name is Debra Meyerson. My name is Debra Meyerson. My name is Debra Meyerson," until, tense with excitement, I lost the melody and timing and the words broke down. By this time, I was overcome, tears streaming down my face. I could say my name again.

· · ·

When it comes to stroke, "There is no cure," wrote Professor Sharon Kaufman in *Medical Anthropology Quarterly*.[8] "Medical knowledge is not authoritative about the long-term care of stroke patients." Once a survivor's stroke is stable, no doctor or rehab therapist can give a particularly accurate forecast of what functional recovery is likely, or possible. Even with extremely detailed images showing where brain damage has occurred, and lots of past history to draw from, every stroke is different. So, survivors approach their recovery with an extremely uncertain path, timeline, and ultimate destination.

The nature of a stroke is particularly damaging to our sense of self. It frequently strikes without warning. The cause is often unknown, random, and unpreventable. It diminishes our ability to decide what type of care to get in the immediate aftermath. And how fast and how much we will recover is often a black box that only time and trust can unlock. Stroke takes away our implicit trust that things happen for a reason, that there are predictors and signs preceding a medical catastrophe, that recovery will follow a certain path. Each time I woke up in my hospital bed, I had a renewed sense of confusion.

In a study of chronic illness, Professor Sharon Kaufman described the feelings of patients recovering from trauma and its impact on their self-image. She observed that for many stroke patients, "The inability of the self to master the body was interpreted as a 'failure' and 'frightening:' it fundamentally shatters the individual's sense of control over the environment."[9]

Former Intel exec Sean Maloney was also taken by ambulance to Stanford Hospital after his stroke. Like mine, Sean's stroke wiped out his ability to write, to speak, and to move his right side. Many years after his stroke, having regained much but not all of those capabilities, he described the shattering loss of wholeness and control he experienced shortly after his stroke. "I had this jarring recognition that everything can fail."

Stroke survivors are often warned that progress will be slow, with occasional jumps forward as well as some steps back. Even knowing this, every step back brings concern that there has been more damage or additional stroke activity. And any new stroke could be life-threatening. It begins to feel as if you're living on a precipice. Said Andrea Helft: "I was really afraid. I was afraid it was going to happen again . . . any time I felt any sort of big emotion, I would think, 'Oh no, I'm killing myself, because it's going to happen again.'"

· · ·

About two weeks after I'd arrived at Santa Clara Valley Medical Center, I'd continued to make progress. With support, I could walk down the hall, and while speech was still far from fluent, I was able to communicate far more. The doctors thought I'd be ready to go home in a few days.

One morning, while still at the Valley Medical rehab program, Steve and I began what had become our on-the-way-to-breakfast therapy game. He would point to objects, and I would name them. But this morning was different: words that I could speak the day before were garbled. Much of the limited speech I had regained was gone. He found the doctor, and an immediate CT scan confirmed that I had experienced another stroke.

We were devastated. The words I'd spoken less than twenty-four hours before and all the phrases I'd practiced were once again inaccessible. I tried desperately to speak some sentences to prove to Steve, to the medical staff, and most of all to myself, that everything was OK. But the words just wouldn't come out. I was moved back to Stanford Hospital.

Fortunately, I hadn't lost any of the physical strength and movement I had regained, but this second stroke was in one of the main speech centers of the brain. And it was bad. More brain tissue killed and more speech function lost. This second stroke was caused by a blood clot that had formed behind the same flap of tissue that caused the first stroke. They expected that the medication I was taking—blood thinners, anticlotting drugs, and blood pressure elevators—would help the flap reattach to the artery wall so clots couldn't form there. But, as with the initial dissection, my body seemed to be an anomaly and the widely accepted "standard of care" didn't work for me.

Back at Stanford, my situation worsened. In addition to the new stroke, my blood pressure dropped and my platelet level plummeted. So, once again, I was moved to the ICU. Unlike my first ICU experience, I was completely coherent this time and furious about my slide. I had learned that it was best to do as much therapy as soon as possible, so completely frustrated that the ICU at Stanford does not offer much therapy. With Steve's insistence, and a bit of creativity, we tried to continue as much rehab activity as possible to help lessen the feeling of setback. Steve wrote in a CaringBridge entry:

> *To once again use the "two steps forward, one step back" framing: if it's 100 steps for Deb to get back to normal, it feels like we had taken about ten steps forward from the post stroke low, and have now fallen five or six back. I so wish it was better, but am thankful that it's not even worse.*

A week into my second stay in the ICU, Adam and Steve were walking me through a series of exercises. For the snow angel, I had to move my weakened right leg out to the side and back. After ten reps, Steve asked me if I could do the same with my unaffected left leg. I swung it out with such force that I knocked Adam off the side of the bed. Next, they asked me if I could lift my right leg off the bed: my inability to do this the day before had concerned the neurologist and led to another MRI. But now I gritted my teeth and gave it everything I had, lifting my leg a good eight inches off the bed. I held it as long as I could, maybe five seconds. Steve and Adam's hoots and hollers brought the nurses running, but they saw from my clenched grin that there was nothing to worry about.

Soon after, Danny picked up a bundle of information sheets that the speech therapist had left. I reached across with my good left hand and grabbed it from him. I was still unable to make a sound, but there was work to do, and I was determined that I would be out of the hospital and back teaching in two weeks. I hadn't accepted the fact that I could no longer speak and didn't know what was causing my repeated strokes. In my mind, I was still Professor Meyerson.

· · ·

After much consideration and observation, the doctors told Steve they thought it might be best to perform a surgical procedure. Because of the two unusual events, they were concerned about my blood vessels' behavior and wanted to insert a stent in the artery leading to my brain. A stent is a small, expanding tube that gets threaded through the affected artery all the way to the location of the dissection. Once in place, it expands and physically holds the flap against the artery wall. While the odds of a complication were low, there was a very small risk of puncturing the artery, and that could be fatal; this was in the brain, after all.

We debated the decision. The risk seemed huge. One surgeon helped us frame the situation, "It's not introducing risk. There is risk either way, surgery or no surgery. You're choosing which risk to accept, and we strongly believe this is the lesser risk." We opted for surgery.

The doctors told my family the procedure should take two to three hours. They waited outside the operating room for five hours without word. Pacing the halls, guessing that only a complication could keep things dragging on with no reassurance from the doctor, they feared the worst. Steve, Danny, Aaron and my mom tried to comfort each other, but they also voiced their fears.

Thankfully, I just had blood vessels that were especially complicated to navigate. The operation caused a small nick in a blood vessel, but that healed quickly, and overall, it was a success. After a few days of recovery and observation, I was cleared for rehab at Valley Medical Center, again.

. . .

Shortly after my return to "Valley," as we called it, Danny was coming for another visit. Steve had left thirty minutes before he arrived. Danny made the now familiar journey up to the second floor and down a long hallway to the very end, where I was lucky to have a double room to myself. He walked in and found me face down on the floor, alone, unable to move, a couple of feet from my wheelchair. Panicked, he screamed for help and ran to me. I tried to tell him I was fine, pushing him away and repeating the only word in my vocabulary at the time: a frantic "no, no, no!"

Fortunately, I *was* fine. Danny and the nurses pulled me up and back into my wheelchair and started the now-routine game of twenty questions to find out what had happened. "Did you fall?" "No," I said, but clearly meant yes. "How?" No response. "Did you try to get up by yourself?" asked the nurse. "No," I lied. "What happened to the belt?" Danny pointed to the seat belt, just like a simple lap belt in a car or plane, that was now fastened around my waist. I had a hard time looking him in the eye, and I had a look on my face that my family tells me was increasingly frequent during that phase of my recovery—part grimace and part smirk. It reflected my overwhelming feeling at the time: I was pissed off about my condition and was not about to be told I couldn't do what I wanted to do.

Stuck in the wheelchair and refusing to accept my own condition, I had taken advantage of the brief window when family and nurses were gone. I simply tried to get up and walk away on my own. Of course, I immediately fell flat on my face. I was unable to call for help and couldn't move myself. So Danny walked in and found me on the floor. Once the scare was past, we laughed about it. And we still do—it was an early, clear symbol that my stroke had not robbed me of my stubbornness and determination. Although this episode had no bad consequences, the combination of denial and determination certainly could have ended badly.

In the early days and weeks of my recovery, though I could not speak or move some parts of my body, it did not register with me that this condition might persist beyond those weeks into months or even years. I gradually admitted to myself that I might miss fall quarter at school, but nothing beyond that. If I applied all my willpower to pushing back, surely I could overpower this failure of my body.

All my life, I had worked hard to achieve the things I cared about, and generally did so without much help. Academics. Sports. Fitness. For years I made room for an intense job and attentive parenthood, alongside a spouse I loved who did the same. We both paused our careers for a year to homeschool our kids and live on a sailboat as a family, a dream Steve and I first talked about before we were married. There were hundreds of reasons not to do it, but we figured it out. When a wall stood between me and my goals, I did whatever it took to climb the wall or break through it. It never occurred to me that the stroke would be any different.

A few years later, a college friend of Danny's was going through a shockingly similar situation when his dad suffered a severe stroke. He had been a professor, like me. His stroke was caused by a dissection, like mine. He had lost significant speech, refused to accept his new condition, and just wanted to go back to work. As they exchanged stories, Danny's friend told him about the time he walked into his dad's hospital room only to find his father on the floor next to his wheelchair, unable to move, and unwilling to admit he'd just tried to get up and walk away from his new reality. Same story.

Like me, he had not yet come to terms with his new situation. He fully understood who he was and what he did prior to his stroke. Like me, he assumed he would quickly reenter his old life, clinging tightly to the person he used to be. This determination is critical in many ways, driving us to work hard at therapy and to make progress faster and longer than many professionals in the field tell us we can. But it also highlights what can be an unrealistic and emotionally counterproductive single-minded focus on our past selves.

In the early period after stroke, many of us struggle to process our new condition. We have not accepted our lack of control over our situation. We have not faced up to our reduced capabilities and loss of independence. Although denial and determination can aid in our rehab, they can also shut us off from understanding other interpretations of recovery, where returning to our past capabilities is incomplete. Early in my recovery, I—like so many others I've gotten to know—had not yet started to wrestle with my changing identities because I was still stubbornly clinging to the old ones.

This is not the case for everyone. Like everything else in stroke, each of us experiences our shift in self-image in our own way. In *A Stitch of Time*, Lauren Marks described an early experience of stroke that was completely different from mine. She wrote:

> *I had woken up from brain surgery changed—there was me, here and now, but I sensed there was another shadowy character in the mix here, too: The Girl I Used to Be. I couldn't easily access the memories of this girl in any complete way and wasn't actively engaging in her senses of attachment or desire. I didn't know if I wanted what she used to want, or if I cared about what she used to care about. And, strangely enough, I wasn't mourning the loss of that past self. She was simply gone, which was neither a good nor a bad thing.*[10]

Regardless of timing, though, ultimately we all face a similar journey. One day, we know who we are. Our various identities are fairly clear and aligned, not even a cause for thought. We might change and grow over time, but at each moment, we know who we fundamentally are. In an instant, this is upended. Some, like me, are in complete denial for quite a while. Others understand and accept their situation much more quickly and, therefore, start thinking far sooner than I did about the incongruity between who they were and who they now are. Eventually, we all come to appreciate that many of the qualities we have defined ourselves by are now threatened by our loss of capabilities. A mother who cannot hold her child's hand. A sailor with no sense of balance. A baseball player who cannot throw. Or in my case, a teacher without words.

CHAPTER 3.

A Teacher without Words

The second sentence of my 2001 book, *Tempered Radicals*, asks, "How do members of an organization express identities and values that are different from the majority culture while fitting into that culture?"[11] For years, I had studied how people can effectively align their internal selves—how they define themselves—with the roles they play and the environments in which they play them. My work explored how people drew on different parts of their identities—their gender, race, attitudes, and values—to define and shape the world around them. I spent time on an oil rig, living in one of the most macho cultures imaginable, working with a leader who coaxed his men to be more vulnerable and communicative to make sure they stayed safe. I worked with feminist surgeons trying to balance what it meant to specialize in the male-dominated surgery profession with what it meant to her to be a woman.

Even those who study identity academically have trouble defining the term, and they often don't agree with one another. Psychologist Erik Erikson, famous for his theory on psychological development, wrote, "The more one writes about this [identity], the more the word becomes a term for something that is as unfathomable as it is all-pervasive."[12] Often, we think of ourselves as having a single, all-encompassing identity. This isn't how we actually live our lives, though.

Identity is multiple, dynamic, relationship-based, and interpretive. We are constantly evolving, and so are our identities, both informing our choices in life and being informed by them. We each hold many values and exist in many contexts and dimensions that shape our lives, and so we all have various identities that are constantly interacting. Writers and educators Sharon Anderson and Kyle Whitfield offer a definition based not on what identity is but how it's constructed: "Personal identity is developed within social transactions where self-perceptions and possible identities are negotiated with others."[13]

We live in a complex, ever-changing world. To help ourselves navigate this, we create narratives and generalities that give our path through life coherence. Among these are our senses of identity. It is not feasible that, given the complexity of our lives, we would have one single, holistic identity. As Walt Whitman said, "Do I contradict myself? Very well, I contradict myself. I am large, I contain multitudes." It is inevitable that we will have a dynamic sense of identity, carved in various contexts and relationships.

Psychology research has shown repeatedly and powerfully that harmony among our various identities can be emotionally beneficial.[14] When there is no clash between how we think of ourselves and how we present ourselves in various situations, we are happier and more resilient. If there is a disparity, we become stressed or even distressed. Sometimes, we encounter this in relatively subtle situations. How do you proceed when a colleague that you consider a friend is not performing? What do you do when an important and unforeseen need at work would force you to break a family commitment? Do you dress according to professional norms or in the attire you find expresses yourself and keeps you comfortable?

These decisions, even seemingly minor ones, stress us because we are trying to simultaneously live in accordance with two identities that are both important to us but which clash. We all deal with these situations of competing identity, though often in fairly mild ways and without realizing it.

My stroke took this dissonance to a whole new level. "Brains give rise to our ability to form relationships and make life meaningful. Sometimes, they break," wrote neurosurgeon Paul Kalanithi in his bestselling autobiography,

When Breath Becomes Air.[15] Along with destroying brain tissue, stroke can obliterate the continuity of the narrative we've constructed around the activities, relationships, and aspirations we've spent our lives building. It made me feel that many of the things I define myself by were now false.

I'm a professor, yet I cannot speak. I'm independent, yet I need a tube to eat. I'm an athlete, yet I cannot walk without support. I'm a mother, yet my kids are comforting me. I'm healthy and active, yet I'm stuck in the ICU. Before we recover or rebuild, we are left mostly alone to face an image of self we no longer measure up to. Dr. Kerry Kuluski and her colleagues from the Institute of Health Policy at University of Toronto describe this as a "discredited notion of self."[16]

• • •

Emmanuel "Manny" Gigante was a hard-charging systems engineer in the Bay Area. "It was 2003, so I was deeply immersed in the dot-com culture, that very fast-paced, high-pressure environment. I was working twenty-hour days, basically," he told me. Manny was the head of a large Filipino family. His mother is one of thirteen siblings, and they all have kids and grandkids living in the United States. When he was twenty-nine, blood coagulated in his brain and caused a massive stroke.

His large family meant he had a tremendous amount of family support. But the man of the house was expected to be the strong leader, and he had a tough time reconciling this expectation with his physical disabilities after his stroke. His mom had trouble seeing him as the head of the family now, and he had trouble seeing himself as a man.

"Initially, I really struggled with the whole thing where the father's role is supposed to be machismo—go play sports with my son, throw the ball around, shoot baskets," he said. Most startlingly, Manny lost his first son, three days away from celebrating his fifth birthday, in an accident two

years after his stroke. He told me that he can't count the number of times
he's asked himself, "Would that have happened differently if I was able-
bodied?" Could he have reacted more quickly and prevented the accident?
More generally, he questioned whether he could be an effective father in
a wheelchair. He was forced to reexamine everything about the ways he
previously defined himself, and that wasn't easy.

I was stubborn about confronting the changes in my life. It wasn't until
three years after my stroke, forced to give up my professorship at Stanford,
that I reluctantly had to accept that full physical and speech recovery
might never happen for me. Until that moment, I had worked furiously to
recover my old life, and returning to teaching was a critical part of that. My
vocation wasn't just a job to me. I had spent a huge part of my life creating
and spreading knowledge about social issues around diversity, gender, and
identity. I cared deeply about these topics, had built expertise and reputation
in them, and worked my ass off to carve out a career researching and
teaching them full time. The tempered radicals I worked with inspired me
with their commitment, clear-headed belief in a cause, and ability to balance
multiple goals. I had grown to consider myself part of that community.

A huge piece of my own identity was derived from this. I had trouble
coping with losing this, even short-term, and had refused to think about
losing it more permanently. The realization that I could no longer be part
of that world was a new trauma. "One of the reasons that trauma is so
devastating is because of its impact on individuals' beliefs about who they
are and who they can become," wrote my friend and colleague Sally Maitlis,
an identity expert and professor of organizational behavior at Oxford. "The
negative emotion generated by a trauma signals the loss of or damage to a
significant aspect of self."[17]

Complex and scary emotions started swirling in my head at about
this time. I started to ask myself, explicitly but silently, whether I had lost
essential parts of life. I was not a tenured professor anymore and probably

never would be again. I was not a fully able-bodied person. Would I be able to sail and ski again? Would family vacations be limited to comfortable road trips rather than new adventures? I was committed to keep working on my recovery and believed I would keep getting better (and I have). But I started, ever so slowly, to accept that all the work in the world might not get my old life back. And I began to wonder, "If that is the case, who am I now?"

A chapter in *Tempered Radicals* is titled "Turning Personal Threats into Opportunities." The first section of the chapter is called "Recognizing Choice." It deals with ways to escape feeling trapped by a difficult situation and develop other responses and perspectives. It can be hard, especially when the situation seems hopeless, but the people and organizations I studied had provided many examples of how it could be done. One of the strategies described was *Seeing the Complex Self.* Nine years before my stroke, I wrote, "It is important to remember that we can evaluate other aspects of the situation and choose how best to respond rather than feeling forced to defend a singular 'true self.'"[18]

I started to realize I had been asking the wrong question. I was evaluating my future against the identities I had built for myself based on the past. Maybe I needed to look at myself a bit more deeply. Not only my capabilities and what I had done but more fundamentally my values and what I really cared about. My identities lived not just in my accomplishments but also in the underlying drives that pushed me toward them in the first place. Rather than "Who am I now?" I could choose to ask myself a different question: "Who do I *want* to be now?"

· · ·

I had spent my career trying to help people understand how to make sense of their place in a chaotic, complex world. This is achieved not by finding the one true self but by reaching a more complex understanding of how our many selves interact with the world around us. As psychology professor Kenneth Gergen put it, "One's identity is continuously emergent, re-formed, and redirected as one moves through the sea of ever-changing relationships. In the case of 'Who am I?' it is a teeming world of provisional possibilities."[19] Well into my poststroke recovery, I was starting to remember some of the critical things about identity that I had known, in a much more impersonal way, before.

Four years after my stroke, I had the pleasure of meeting Lakshmi Ramarajan, a leading identity scholar from Harvard Business School. I had long admired her work, and we were both attending a gender conference at Harvard organized by our mutual friend Robin Ely, also a professor there. Lakshmi was patient with my slow and difficult speech. Reacting to my early thoughts, she explained that her work had taught her that a person can have many identities or self-definitions at once. These are made up of an ever-changing mix of attributes such as organizational membership, profession, gender, ethnicity, religion, nation, and family roles.[20] Lakshmi embraces the view that identity is not one dominant view of ourselves but rather the network of meanings we hold in multiple contexts such as group membership, role, or characteristics.[21] She has surveyed the literature in five different fields and studied the hierarchies and relationships they use to define identity. Although there are many similarities among these fields, there are significant disagreements as well.

In my quest to understand my own evolving life, I certainly was not going to try to bridge half a dozen academic disciplines to resolve the puzzle of defining identity. But I realized that I didn't need to. I needed to find a deeper understanding of my own poststroke identity and set myself on a path toward rebuilding a life aligned to that. This wouldn't be easy, but in my poststroke life of therapy, three grown kids, and a gap where my career had been, I had the time, training, and reason to examine my life in a way I never had before. What clashes and gaps and moments were causing me the most anguish, and why? What values did I hold most dear and how could I live those out, perhaps in a different way? What communities, achievements, roles, and feelings did I find most fulfilling, and how could I build my life around them? I may never be able to answer these questions completely, but I have found many tools and lessons that have proved helpful.

• • •

What makes a fulfilling life? Since its publication in 1943, psychologist Abraham Maslow's famous Hierarchy of Needs has been the basis for many investigations into human needs, desires, motivation, and behavior. The pyramid arranges what humans care about, what ultimately generates a fulfilling life, as a hierarchy: once a lower level is satisfied, then and only then can a person be motivated by the next set of needs.

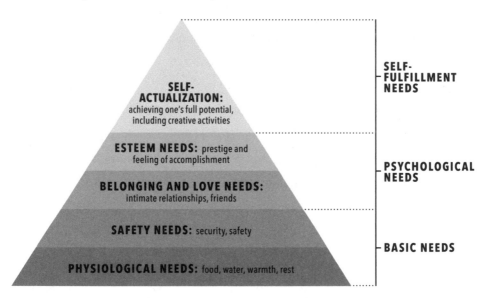

The empirical and theoretical validity of Maslow's hierarchy is hotly debated, but it's certainly a useful tool for thinking about my problem. Maslow's hierarchy gave me a way to understand my desires, frustrations, and challenges—both physical and emotional. There were needs that I could articulate and others that were less obvious, even to me.[22]

BASIC NEEDS: Physiological needs clearly came first. I needed acute medical care. I was completely dependent on others to keep me alive. Since my survival was in doubt, little else mattered. **Safety needs** came next: I was reliant on others for basic security. Like other survivors, I strongly resented my dependence, and this was a cause of massive frustration. Regaining the ability to provide for my own basic needs was an early motivator.

PSYCHOLOGICAL NEEDS: A desire to belong accelerated my poststroke identity crisis. Loss of language was a big issue here, creating gaps within previous relationships and communities. Even once I felt secure and embraced by family and friends, I lacked **self-esteem,** and my previous avenues to build it had closed. I could not teach, ski, or even be a mother as I used to.

SELF-FULFILLMENT: As I came to realize that my abilities and options in life were forever changed, the real challenge presented itself. How could I now achieve **self-actualization?** How could I grow as a person when I was now so far removed from the person I had been working on for fifty-three years? My stroke had thrown me off the path I was on, and I had to find a new one.

This model helped me focus my attention on building a life I wanted, disabilities included. My relationships have changed. Many are harder, some are stronger than ever, and I've developed some incredibly rewarding new ones. My roles and work have changed. I cannot do the teaching I loved, but I've found a new calling in stroke activism, including writing this book and working with nonprofits. My communities are different—fewer

Stanford panels, more stroke conferences. My accomplishments no longer register in academic journals, but I'm frequently told I inspire my friends and family with the obstacles I have overcome. I don't advise students, but I may be a more supportive friend, advocate, and ally than before. I am no longer a tenured professor at a top university, but I can still build and share knowledge in a way that improves others' lives.

CHAPTER 4.

Moving Forward

Four years after my stroke, with choppy speech starting to return, I was offered the opportunity to address a group of stroke survivors, doctors, therapists, and advocates at a Pacific Stroke Association event. I was interested but nervous. I used to comfortably address classes, executives, and large conferences about complex organizational topics. Now, I'd be struggling to string together simple sentences. I agreed. This was a small step toward embracing my new life as a stroke survivor. With great effort and a lot of help, I prepared and practiced (and practiced, and practiced) a presentation I called "Lucky to Be Alive." Toward the end of my ten-minute talk, I found myself saying a sentence I hadn't prepared at all: "I am a happier person now."

I've also found myself spontaneously saying, "Life sucks." There are certainly moments and days when it is a little hard to appreciate my good fortune. Eight years after my stroke, I was in Tahoe with family working on this book, and I found myself in a particularly bad place. I posted on my blog, "I don't think it's realistic for most survivors to ever stop mourning the loss of the life that was, at least from time to time. I've spent the past week on a writing retreat for my book and am really hating how much help I need with it. So I guess I'm really mourning that loss right now." Both states of mind are true. Sometimes I mourn the loss of my old self and feel like life sucks. Other times, I genuinely feel like a happier person than I was before my stroke.

Why are the up-and-down moments so extreme when our situations basically stay the same? Philosophers in ancient Greece (and many since) preached that our emotions are caused not by external situations but by our own internal interpretations of them. We are not sad because it's raining: we are sad because we have let ourselves be upset that it's raining. To at least some degree, this is a choice to be upset rather than happy with rain. To at least some degree, the reason I get depressed isn't because I have limited communication and don't have use of my arm; I get depressed because I'm remembering all the things I could do before my stroke that are no longer accessible to me and comparing to that.

Health researchers Dr. Kuluski and her colleagues call this process "narrative reconstruction." In chronic illness, they say that there are three common frames of mind:

THE CHAOS NARRATIVE, characterized by a loss of hope

THE RESTITUTION NARRATIVE, characterized by a focus on recovery

THE QUEST NARRATIVE, characterized by the belief that illness is an opportunity for growth.[23]

The narrative we tell ourselves and others dramatically influences how we act. We are not stuck in one narrative, nor is it always a choice. Sometimes, I can't help but focus on the loss (and the chaos it has created). Other times, I zero in on restitution, with complete determination to focus on physical or speech recovery. And during some periods, I revel in the newfound perspective this experience has brought me, and the work I am doing to understand my own life better and to help other stroke survivors. I often feel optimistic about recovery one day and then feel completely hopeless the next. But understanding that we have some agency in choosing our narrative has helped me stay in the quest frame of mind more often, and I dig myself out of chaos a bit quicker.

In *Option B: Facing Adversity, Building Resilience, and Finding Joy*, Sheryl Sandberg, COO of Facebook, and coauthor Adam Grant, psychologist and professor at the Wharton School of Business, write powerfully of Sheryl's loss of her husband in an instant to a cardiac arrhythmia, and her journey to move through grief and bounce back. She quotes Allen Rucker, who wrote about his experience of paralysis, "I won't make your skin crawl by saying it's a blessing in disguise. It's not a blessing, and there is no disguise. But there are things to be gained and things to be lost, and on certain days I'm not sure that the gains are not as great as, or even greater than, the inevitable losses." Resilience—the strength and speed of our response to adversity—isn't something we simply have or don't have; it's something we can build and reinforce.[24]

In my low moments, I doubt my resilience. I have committed myself to remodeling my life for the future, but sometimes I cannot help but look back at what I've lost and despair. However, I've tried to get better at recognizing which narrative I'm in and adjusting accordingly. Doing so has helped me control my emotions more consistently, build resilience, and create solutions and improvements in this adverse situation.

I've developed three major strategies that have been particularly helpful as I rebuild my life and my identity. As will be seen in the next section of the book, they are echoed by many other survivors in nearly every aspect of our poststroke journeys.

LOOK FORWARD, NOT BACK: It can be hard to do. I often slip. But reminding myself to look ahead and focus on progressive small wins in the future rather than comparisons to the past is key to continued progress.

FOCUS ON DEEPER VALUES: Drawing on what I care most about, whether family or fitness or advocacy—or for many, religion or a cause—is not only a source for motivation but a way to guide my actions. Knowing what matters most helps me set goals that I can work toward, care about, and achieve— whether that's publishing a book or swimming independently.

SEEK OPPORTUNITIES FOR GROWTH: Healthy or not, there are always infinite opportunities for us to become more mature, complex, meaningful people. Growth that is exciting and even novel—like letting go of my career stress—makes my progress more than just clawing back what I've lost, it's deeply rewarding.

I probably will never stop being frustrated by my lost abilities. But I am moving forward. I am rebuilding a very full and rewarding life despite my loss. As Sandberg relates hearing from a friend about grieving the loss of a loved one: you never get over it, but you can get past it.

• • •

LOOK FORWARD, NOT BACK

Julia Fox Garrison, a stroke survivor and now a stroke activist, admits that she may never fully recover all of her capabilities, but she will never give up trying. There is a reason that those of us recovering from strokes refer to ourselves as survivors rather than victims. "There's a victim, and there's a survivor, and it's a true choice," she explained. "A victim doesn't thrive, survivors do." It's not just a cheerier, more optimistic outlook. Focusing on continuous improvement rather than on what was lost leads to better results, both in terms of measurable improvement and in quality of life. Fox Garrison said, "The paramount thing is your attitude. That's 90 percent of your recovery. If your attitude is good, you're going to have a better outcome."

There are plenty of times I feel fed up with my immobile hand, my limping walk, and my difficult speech. Taken as a whole, they remind me of how far I am from my old, complete self. But those around me tell me they see huge improvements over time, and when I successfully concentrate on the task at hand—keeping my foot balanced as I walk, which I couldn't do last year, or talking more smoothly than I used to late at night—then I can see the progress I am making, too.

In *Tempered Radicals*, I wrote about the value of small wins, a concept developed by organizational theorist Karl Weick, a colleague and coauthor. Small wins are seemingly little victories that have a large impact on how we perceive our situation. Weick studied people in frustrating circumstances where they could feel overwhelmed and helpless. When they set goals and focused on small wins, however, they found that, over time, the wins piled up and created meaningful change in how they felt about the situation. "A small win reduces importance ('this is no big deal'), reduces demands ('that's all that needs to be done'), and raises perceived skill levels ('I can do at least that')," wrote Weick.[25] Breaking down big goals into manageable bits makes the task at hand less daunting and more achievable.

Focusing on small wins is *hard*.[26] And to do it all the time is impossible. I constantly find myself looking at the large gap of what I've lost, rather than the small next step forward I can take. This is OK. It's inevitable, and we must give ourselves permission to be frustrated, imperfect, and even to grieve.

Stroke can be especially cruel because it doesn't feel like anything should be wrong. This is particularly true for those of us with aphasia. I can voice my ideas in my head; I just can't get them out for others to hear. That disconnect, the fact that many of us are all there inside but are not able to express ourselves to the outside, is a constant reminder of what we used to be. So, of course, we can't help but mourn our past selves from time to time.

Sheryl Sandberg and Adam Grant write of a strategy for these moments—leaning into the suck. Think about all the things that suck, about how bad it is . . . and then think about how much worse it could have been.[27] I could easily be dead, and in past decades probably would have been. I could have lost all movement and all speech, like many stroke survivors I've met. This could have happened to one of my children instead of me. I could be battling this alone, rather than with a dedicated family, a support network, and financial security. I am luckier than most in this respect, but all of us survivors can think of ways our situation could be worse, and so we have things to be thankful for. After leaning into the suck, the comparisons to my past recede and are replaced by comparisons to worse alternatives, and I can again see my blessings more clearly. And with that clarity, I can focus on what I value in my life and set attainable goals for the future.

Our ability to adapt as humans is truly remarkable. An incredibly powerful example is a concept known as the hedonic treadmill, first studied as hedonic adaptation by psychologists Brickman and Campbell in 1971.[28] The theory says that two people can be equally happy today, and if tomorrow one wins the lottery and one wakes up paraplegic, they will diverge sharply in happiness. But six months later, they will be back to equal. The lottery winner comes back to neutral, and so does the person with severe disabilities.[29] What matters is not some absolute level of satisfaction but rather how our reality compares with our expectations. We are wired to adapt, and our happiness can follow.

Immediately after his stroke, Mark Wells was bitter and thought, "I'm better off dead." But before long, he found inspiration in several places. On a TV program, he heard a female preacher say, "You've just got to keep praising [God], because, one day, your body will catch up to the praise." That was a trigger that helped him look forward a bit, and he calls it a turning point. He started to look at his situation in a different way. "You know what," he told me, "I just got to learn how to be content." People tell him there are others far worse off, and he sees this and is thankful. At the same time, he knows, "There are a lot of people that are doing well, too, and I want to be doing well." He uses this attitude to battle through constant discomfort and look ahead.

• • •

FOCUS ON DEEPER VALUES

Julia Fox Garrison said there was a big turning point for her when she realized she was trying to be pre-stroke Julia, and that person could never be. The realization opened the door to creating a new identity for herself. There are things she lost that she loved, like her physicality, but she continually asks herself, "How do you change something that you love and make something else new, introduce new things into your life that can bring you joy?" Like many of us survivors, she discovered that recovery does not have to mean rebuilding exactly what was lost. In the face of dramatic change, it is particularly helpful to rethink our assumptions and discover their underlying principles. We often assume we know why we value the things we've always cared about. But often, we've never actually broken them down to the core and figured out why they are so important. Recovery doesn't have to mean regaining all your lost capabilities. It doesn't have to mean returning to your prior job. For Julia, it has been rebuilding a life of meaning and joy.

Karl Weick, the social scientist who coined the term "small wins," also introduced the concept of sensemaking into organizational studies, another idea that I've drawn on in my previous work. Sensemaking is the "activity of framing experienced situations as meaningful," describes Weick. It is something we do both consciously and unconsciously all the time. Weick identified seven properties of sensemaking, the very first of which is identity: who people think they are shapes how they interpret events and react to them.[30] The processes of defining ourselves and finding meaning externally are deeply intertwined, and this is demonstrated in the journeys of many stroke survivors.

Sally Maitlis has studied trauma recovery and has seen the importance of sensemaking in people's recovery and post-trauma life. She points to positive identity, which she said includes an understanding of one's strengths and resourcefulness in the face of adversity, and an appreciation of one's ability to transcend deep pain.[31] Our setbacks provide us with a chance to build resilience, discover new or previously untapped strength, and define our meaning anew. If we can use our situation as an opportunity to take stock of our deeper values and grow them, we have adopted a motivational force to drive us during the good times and the bad. For some this is faith; for others, family. For many that I've met, it has become stroke activism. For a few, it's golf.

In Maslow's hierarchy of needs, the top of the pyramid is self-actualization. The questions we face in this process are not unique to trauma victims. It's the same search for meaning that many feel when they are relatively healthy and grief-free. A stroke (or other setback) may redefine our potential in ways that leave a gap—we may no longer be able to use our old methods for achieving self-actualization. But we are still searching for purpose just like everyone else. The adversity caused by the trauma and capability gap can force valuable self-reflection. As Maitlis writes, "In the struggle to come to terms with the new reality that follows a trauma, people are forced to give up certain assumptions and goals and to create new meanings and a new understanding of the world and their place in it. This process is both confusing and painful but contains the opportunity for significant change."[32] If we let it, our trauma can be an opportunity for sensemaking and can inspire us to be more deliberate in choosing how to live a fulfilled life.

Laure Wang was cofounder of Asia Alternatives, a former vice president at Goldman Sachs, an alumna of Stanford University and Harvard Business School, and mother of two sons. While at a meeting in Hong Kong, Laure fainted and was rushed to the hospital. After several days of fighting for her life, Laure was diagnosed as having suffered a severe brain-stem stroke. At age thirty-nine, it left her with locked-in syndrome—she was aware and awake but unable to move anything except her eyes. She was initially overwhelmed with sadness, self-pity, and depression. She felt that life was only worth living for the sake of her husband and their two children. "But because of my faith," she wrote, "I made it through my suffering by becoming stronger and better. I could have become bitter and victimized. But because I knew I was loved by God, I had hope and a positive mentality." She now uses an alphabet board and eye movements to spell out the words she wants to say, and she wrote that in her book, *Reflections on a Changed Life.*[33]

Mark Davis was a self-proclaimed workaholic, toiling long hours in multiple jobs as soon as he was old enough to start working. Owner of a string of rental properties across the bay from San Francisco, he never slowed down enough to reflect on life. Then he suffered a stroke and all of his constant running around came to a screeching halt. "I feel like life, the universe, or whatever sits you down does it for a reason," Mark told me. "You have a different way of looking at life after everything's said and done." Mark's stroke gave him time, which he used to explore his history, his beliefs, and the way his identity was constructed. Gaining a deeper understanding of his African-American heritage has been a huge learning experience for him, and he has a new sense of pride as a result.

Many of the survivors I've met have been inspired by their greater understanding of life with disabilities and the desire to help others who live with them. Like several other survivors I spoke to, Kathy Howard has found a rewarding life by immersing herself in her identity as a stroke survivor. "Before my stroke I had some exciting jobs, but I was always looking for something," she told me. "I had a stroke and now I've found it." Kathy's mission now is talking with and encouraging new survivors. She said it is her dream job. "I love being able to walk into a room and say, 'You know, I was one of those people who was told I might never walk again, but I *drove* out here to see you.'" Kathy has made significant recovery but still feels almost constant pain and buzzing and burning in her left side. Yet she said she feels more fulfilled in life now than ever before.

• • •

SEEK OPPORTUNITIES FOR GROWTH

"What doesn't kill you makes you stronger." Common in today's pop culture, this phrase was inspired by German philosopher Friedrich Nietzsche, who used a slightly different version in a book published in 1889. He and many other philosophers, psychologists, and scientists have long believed that people do more than survive adversity; we *need* it to thrive.[34] Modern science supports this. Of course, I'm not arguing that stroke survivors can or do emerge more capable than before blood clots or aneurysms wreaked havoc on their brains. But I do strongly believe that strokes, like all traumas and setbacks, are opportunities for real and valuable growth.

People who suffer setbacks recover with strength and resilience if they focus on the critical question, "What can I take away from this?" Without addressing that issue, the potential for despair is real. But commitment to engaging deeply with that question creates the possibility for transformative growth.

In *Option B*, Sandberg and Grant write about three different outcomes that psychologists find in people who have come through trauma. The first result is struggle: some people develop PTSD, depression, anxiety, or difficulty functioning in everyday life. The second possibility is resilience: some people bounce back to the emotional state they were in before the trauma occurred. But finally, there was a third possibility. "People who suffered could 'bounce forward,'" according to Sandberg and Grant.[35] They refer to this bouncing forward as post-traumatic growth.

Five years after my stroke, my father-in-law passed away. My husband, a rock as always, supported his mom, Marjorie, through the loss of her husband of sixty years. Steve drew on our experience of celebrating silver linings and bouncing forward. "You have to let yourself accept that in some ways, your daily life can be better without dad. And that's OK." Marjorie had wanted to redecorate the apartment, but her husband didn't see the need. As she got used to living alone for the first time in her life, she gradually redesigned much of her condo unit to make it her own. Some things would be worse, and she might be lonely. But she could also take liberties she previously did not have and learn to thrive living on her own for the first time in her life, with lots of support. She could go to the theater more, which she loved but had rarely attended since her husband started losing his hearing. She could embrace these opportunities and not feel guilty. Steve was trying to pass on a lesson that we had learned, as have so many others who go through trauma: it's OK to embrace silver linings; they can help point the way to opportunities for learning and growth.

Diane Indelicato and her husband Jim, who suffered a severe stroke, find a lot to be thankful for in the recovery process. "He's so funny now. He laughs. He was so serious before. It's one of the positives, many positives, in my mind," Diane told me. Julia Fox Garrison said her stroke allowed her to cut a lot of negativity from her life. Andrea Helft found a more balanced attitude after her stroke. "I would really like to maintain this . . . I don't even know what to call it. Maybe it's appreciation. I don't want to be back to my old self where I always had my jaw clenched, and my stress level was up to here."

For a very long time, I simply could not acknowledge that anything good could come from my stroke. What good can come from a lack of mobility or an inability to communicate without a game of twenty questions? It all felt so bad—the physical hardship, the emotional struggles, the identity crises, the feelings of dependency, the grief over the loss of a past life . . . all of that sucks. For a long time, I couldn't see past that part of the story.

But what doesn't suck? A calmer demeanor, lower stress about work and accomplishment. A bigger appetite and a greater enjoyment of food. Watching my kids mature into caring adults as they participated in my care. Exceptionally tight relationships with friends who stepped up in incredible ways to support not just me but my family every day for the past eight years. A louder laugh and a bigger sense of humor. An ever-present (well, mostly present) appreciation for my mom and my husband, who have been as dedicated as any family members could be. The closer relationship I had developed with my father-in-law before he passed away, as my aphasia helped me empathize with his hearing troubles. The deepened commitment of my adult kids to family time and closeness. Giving a keynote speech on June 17, 2017, at the Shirley Ryan AbilityLab in Chicago, as part of National Aphasia Awareness Month. It was the most inspiring gathering I've ever been a part of, made so by an amazing community that I didn't even know existed ten years ago.

. . .

"I don't know about you," Kathy Howard said to me in our interview, "but there are still days even eight years out when I think, 'This is just nuts. I'm tired of this. Maybe I don't want to be in this stroke community anymore.'" I agree. There are days when I, too, am tired of all of this. The therapy, the workarounds, the battle with my body, the desire to do more, to be more than my current capabilities allow.

This book has been the hardest thing I've ever done. The challenge to bring together my identities as scholar and stroke survivor has been incredibly painful at times. It has reinforced my ability and my resolve to look forward. But it has also forced me to look back. Back at this journey, back at my old life and capabilities, and back at my last book-writing process, which required so much less help. This has put me face-to-face, every day, with all I've lost. When I feel most cast down by those things, I try to remember the three strategies from this chapter: look forward, focus on deeper values, and seek growth.

It has been almost nine years since my series of strokes in the summer of 2010. After the first months in the hospital, I've been lucky to have no more strokes or major setbacks. But while my initial drama was over, the journey of stroke recovery was just beginning. I've had to find strategies to deal with never-ending therapy and limited speech, to redefine my friendships, families and partnerships, and to change my career and hobbies.

The next section of this book explores each of these slices of poststroke life in detail. In each are pieces of my story, along with more complete stories of what other survivors have experienced and how they managed the change in their lives after stroke. Each of our stories is different, and each of us has found different struggles, silver linings, and strategies to cope and grow. Hearing others' experiences has helped me in every part of my own journey.

The process has made me more convinced than ever that I can rebuild a full life, even if I can't recover all of my past capabilities. I used to think recovery meant a return to pre-stroke living—a full recovery of my speech, use of my right hand, walking and running without a limp. But like the many other survivors in the next section, I've grown to think differently through my poststroke journey. Recovery is building a life of meaning that fulfills my potential, a life that embodies the many aspects of who I am: a loved and loving member of an amazing family, a creator of knowledge, an active woman, a leader in stroke recovery, a stubborn advocate, a grateful friend, and a stroke survivor. I've come to think of recovery in terms of the top of Maslow's pyramid, not the bottom: focusing less on basic needs and regaining capabilities, and more on a quest for meaning and growth.

PART TWO:

WHAT IT'S REALLY LIKE,

Outside and Inside

CHAPTER 5.

The Grind of Therapy

Four months after my stroke, my family gathered for the winter holiday. During breakfast at a restaurant one morning, they struggled to remember the name of the popular movie about a pig that was trained to herd sheep. As everyone else fumbled unsuccessfully through their memories, I suddenly blurted out, "Babe!"

All heads whipped around to look at me. I looked astonished. They were beaming. Steve began hooting, and everyone started high-fiving me and each other. "Babe" was the first unprompted word I had spoken since my stroke. I had regained about twenty words through practiced therapy and repetition, but this was the first original thought to pass my lips in months.

Unfortunately, those breakthrough moments are rare. After eight years of daily effort and countless hours of work, I've had maybe ten dramatic breakthroughs, but progress has been steady. I can now generally find the words I need to get across a simple message, but not always. I cannot share the more complex thoughts I still carry in my brain.

My physical recovery has been equally meaningful and excruciatingly slow. Often, I do not even notice my own improvements until somebody I have not seen in a while points them out. But when I look back on the past eight years or even the past three, I can see the tremendous improvement. I now have relatively good mobility but walk with a limp and still have no functional use of my right hand. I have days when my leg is a little looser or words come a little easier, and others when my recent gains seem to recede.

The term "recovery" is often used after strokes, and it's a word that can evoke thoughts of rest—passively letting the body heal. However, real gains come not just from time and rest but from rigorous work and training. For most stroke survivors, this means hours of physical, speech, and occupational therapy. We fight through the physical and verbal challenges of daily life, including the slow conversations interrupted by "No, say it right" from family members.

Rehab is a full-time commitment after stroke, and even when a full recovery becomes unlikely (if not impossible), therapy continues because incremental improvements are still worth fighting for. It is a grind; it is frustrating; and, at times, the slow rate of improvement does not seem worth the effort. But there are also times of inspiration, markers of progress beyond what you're told to expect, and milestones that open up new levels of independence and keep us moving.

For the eight years since my stroke, my daily schedule has largely been oriented around my intensive therapy: three times per week for each of speech, physical, and occupational therapy. That's just the start, too. Often, my morning begins with thirty to sixty minutes of stretching to get my arm and leg loose and primed for the day. For the first few years, I had nearly daily Skype sessions with my mother to check in and work through speech exercises. When I hung up with her, I would often turn to Rosetta Stone and work my way through more exercises to relearn English.

I wanted to do even more and move faster. The standard three hours per day didn't feel as if it was enough. I wanted to get back to who I was before this nightmare began, so I continued practicing as much as I possibly could. With every new task in therapy, I tried to do even more than the prescribed amount. After my stroke, I wanted nothing more than to power through, work myself nonstop into recovery, and put the experience behind me.

Intel executive Sean Maloney called therapy the hardest full-time job he'd ever had, and he's right in so many ways. For many of us, rehab is still a defining, tireless part of our daily lives for years after our strokes. We must orient our lives around it, making trade-offs between therapy and other parts of life. And recovery is not something we put behind us like a healed injury or mended wound: our recovery becomes part of us, a part of our identity, the way a job is to most people.

• • •

Jim Indelicato spent forty years in the U.S. Air Force and Air National Guard. In the latter, he was in charge of physical fitness, but he took early retirement when the base moved. As a lifelong fixer, he was planning to start his own home-rehabbing business. A thirty-two-time marathoner, Jim has been married to his wife Diane for forty-seven years, and they have been best friends since he was fifteen and she was twelve. Together, they have raised a son and two daughters, and they all live in St. Louis.

On September 16, 2010, Jim was driving his big red Silverado pickup truck with "RUN" on the license plate to help rebuild his mother-in-law's house when he started to lose vision. He pulled the truck over and vomited. His vision briefly recovered, and he drove another mile before he had to pull over and turn the truck off. Five hours later, Jim was in the ICU of St. Anthony's Hospital. He had forgotten how to swallow and was in danger of drowning in his own saliva.

After much confusion, the doctors determined that Jim had a tiny blood clot in his brain stem, the part of the brain that controls basic functions like swallowing and breathing. Six different times while at St. Anthony's, Jim went into respiratory distress, each time for longer than the typical one to two days. The doctors tried multiple types of feeding tubes and respirators, but each had problems. Eventually, they installed a feeding tube that bypassed the throat and sent nutrients straight to the stomach, and they performed a tracheotomy to bring air directly into his throat.

Because he couldn't swallow, saliva had built up in his ears, and he couldn't hear much. That had thrown his balance off so much that he was too dizzy to read what his family wrote to communicate with him. "I think that was when we were at our lowest," said his daughter Joy. Jim spent nine months on a ventilator, then more on a facial ventilator. Joy recalled, "The doctor told us he'd be lucky to ever eat pureed food again."

For the first part of his recovery, Jim focused primarily on physical therapy, intent on getting out of the wheelchair. He joined Paraquad, a physical rehab center, to increase independence. Most people go for an hour or so at a time, but Jim would go for two hours of cardio three days a week. Two years later, he moved from his wheelchair to a walker. After that, he shifted his focus to getting rid of his trach, a breathing tube that goes directly into your throat. Despite skepticism from doctors, Jim began working with a speech therapist who helped him relearn how to swallow. "We think that what helped him trigger the swallow is called vitalstim; they put electrodes on his throat and turn the power up. It helped to get movement started," Joy recalled.

It was slow at first, but Jim was insistent, "Turn it up more, turn it up more." The therapist would say, "He's crazy; the man's crazy." To this day, swallowing is difficult for Jim, but he is able to eat solid foods. He enjoyed his first solid meal four years after his stroke. Next up, was becoming less dependent on the ventilator for breathing. He had sleep apnea, and the ventilator he was using blew the air so hard it woke him up at night. He worked constantly on diaphragm exercises so he could breathe on his own. Four and a half years after his stroke, he got rid of the ventilator. "Now he's just using a BIPAP [a device to reduce sleep apnea]," said Joy. "Another victory," said Jim.

• • •

Not long after I met rehabilitation therapist and educator Waleed Al-Oboudi, whom I've worked with for six years, he explained the process I was in store for:

> *If you break your arm, you know what is going to happen. You know they're going to put a cast on it or do surgery. You know the cast will come off in a number of weeks. With stroke, the whole process is a question mark—what will work, how long it will take, what it will cost, and how much function you expect to get back.*

This makes stroke rehab far harder. Nobody could give me expectations, so I was constantly worried about how my progress stacked up. Was I progressing slowly or quickly? What did it mean for my long-term prognosis? How come my doctors and therapists were being so vague? "No one can say precisely which impairments will disappear completely for an individual or when they will disappear," wrote anthropologist Sharon Kaufman.[36]

Because of the unpredictability, positive thinking is particularly important in stroke rehab. The journey is long and hard, and for many of us it is never-ending. If you look at everything you've lost or everything you have left to do, it's overwhelming. However, if you look with determination and positivity at the next one thing to conquer, recovery seems much more manageable. Jim's focus on the 'small wins' ahead is critical. "I will not tell you you can't," said Jim's neurologist, "because you'll make a fool of me."

My primary care physician Sarah Watson said that studies on attitudes and surgical outcomes supported this, too. "People who are optimistic and confident that things will go well actually do better than those who are really fearful," she said. The power of positive thinking is not only mental; it leads to real physical gains in the recovery process. "I don't think anyone thought you would get the level of language you have now," she told me. "It is remarkable given the amount and location of the damage to your brain."

Orienting around small wins helped me and others battle through the grind of therapy, not just in the first year but beyond. "Whether the goals are lofty or modest, as long as they are meaningful . . . and it is clear how his or her efforts contribute to them, progress toward them can galvanize," wrote Karl Weick about small wins.[37] They aren't just helpful milestones; they are psychologically important. Seeing other survivors and what they have accomplished is an inspiration and a reminder to keep fighting and looking forward to more recovery.[38]

● ● ●

When Sean Maloney lost speech and movement in his right arm after the stroke, he didn't lose his tenacity and seemingly inexhaustible capacity for hard work. Sean describes the first days after his stroke as a cruel transition. On day two, there was dawning recognition that he could not just push through what he calls the "'oh, shit' moment." On day five, he simply decided he had to learn to speak and walk again, whatever that took. Sean would set out for walks up and down the ward. "The doctor came up to me and said, 'I've told you! Do not go out around the ward! Get back to your room!'" Unable to speak any retort, Sean simply laughed. No doctor was going to make him feel helpless or stop him on his path to recovery.

A few weeks after his stroke, Sean heard a doctor telling the rest of his case team that he would never row again. He couldn't speak well enough to argue, but that comment stung. Sean knew very well who he was before his stroke, and he was committed to getting back there. On the way home from the hospital, Sean insisted that his wife stop at his rowing club. He unloaded his shell with one hand and, with lots of help, climbed in. "I had no use of my right arm, so I was pretty much rowing in circles," he told me with a laugh several years later. "But it was important to prove to myself that [losing this sport I loved] was just a doctor's opinion. It was not destiny."[39]

Speech and language pathologist Lisa Levine-Sporer testified to Sean's daunting work ethic. "Sean was probably the most motivated individual I ever worked with. When he decided he was going to get better, he knew he had to do it the Sean way." This laser-like intensity pushed him to make as much progress as possible early on. Like me, Sean was originally focused on regaining all of his lost capabilities.

However, I found that rather than push ever-faster, I actually needed to slow myself down to improve. I needed rest; my brain was recovering from a trauma, after all. And I also needed to focus on deliberate form in my rehab. Every movement was rebuilding signals from my brain to my muscles, and those signals should reflect proper movement if we want healthy recovery. "Science has already determined that when the brain is affected, a tremendous amount of repetition is needed to reorganize," said my therapist Waleed Al-Oboudi, founder of the Neuro-IFRÁH (Integrative Functional Rehabilitation And Habilitation) approach to therapy and a practitioner and educator for more than thirty years. It wasn't just about how many reps I could do; it was about how well I could do them. I needed not just determination but discipline. Steve and I adopted a motto to help keep this goal in mind: "Sometimes you have to go slow to recover fast."

Lisa laughed a little when remembering her progression with Sean. "He started seven days a week, and then he realized that maybe it was OK to drop one day. Then later, maybe it was OK to drop off another day, so it was just Monday through Friday." Like me, he realized that this pace was not sustainable and that total recovery was probably not feasible in a short period, if ever. We needed to regain not just our capabilities but other elements of our lives. Time for friends, family, other activities, vacations, and joy had to be built alongside the rehab. This is a marathon, not a sprint.

• • •

For a long time, the belief in the medical community was that most capability recovery after stroke comes within the first twelve months. Fortunately, this is becoming less prevalent. Jim Indelicato's wife Diane said that they had been told not to expect Jim to recover much more after one to two years. She said, "I'm here to tell you, that's *wrong*." This warning is repeated by many of the survivors in this book who, like Jim, Sean, and me, were warned of the one-year plateau and found it to be a myth. It takes determination and creativity, but progress does not stop after twelve months.

It is true that many of us will never get back to our baseline. This sparks a need to reevaluate what we are working toward. Sharon Kaufman wrote of an "existential awareness of the profound disruption in their lives" when stroke patients she talked with realized their lives may never return to "normal."[40] Why are we working so hard if recovery is impossible? We do come to realize that just because we cannot regain all function does not mean we should work any less hard to rebuild a more independent, stable life.

Once home, Jim still needed intense care. "He had a trach, a GI tube, and slept on a ventilator. They said that any time he closed his eyes, he should be on a ventilator because he might quit breathing or not breathe deep enough," said Diane. "I learned to deep suction." Jim had his trach to aid breathing well into his second year of recovery, and doctors had no plans to remove it. His family found and pushed for a new facial mask ventilator, and although the doctors were skeptical, they agreed to try it. Jim was a little bit confused with the new equipment on the first day, but by the second day, it was clear that it was working. Jim used the new ventilator for several months without a hitch, so well into his second year of recovery, the doctor removed his tracheostomy—a big step to take long after the twelve-month improvement barrier. Step by step, Jim kept progressing until four and a half years after his stroke, he was able to get rid of the ventilator completely.

Jim attributes his breathing improvement to the amount of time he spent exercising post stroke, specifically the diaphragm and core exercises he practiced. At one point during our interview, Diane urged, "Let's show how muscular you are. You're very physical. Come on, come on, let's show off a little here, babe."

Now, Jim motivates the other survivors and therapists at Paraquad to keep pursuing progress. His neurologist asked him how he looked so good, and Jim responded, "I'm doing push-ups—four sets of twenty-five." Diane recalls that the neurologist said, "Jim, I've never met a stroke survivor that has ever done one push-up." He is blessed to have his innate determination, an unbelievably supportive family, and access to great care. He also had a stroke in the worst possible location and lost nearly every function one can lose. "He was worse than any of them," said his neurologist. "But he's fighting."

"Jim, what do you say about what you want on your tombstone?" asked Diane. "Don't let anyone say I'm lazy," he responded. And from all accounts, he's lived up to that. "He has surpassed everything people have said he could do," said Diane. His attitude plays a huge role. He has lost his vision, his balance, his ability to walk, swallow, read, and even breathe. He was in the ICU and on life support for weeks. Many years later, Jim is still extremely limited compared with his former self, but that's not how he sees it. At each step, Jim thinks, "another victory."

THE GRIND OF THERAPY: CHAPTER 5 HIGHLIGHTS

- Recovery is not passive; it's incredibly active.
- It will be the hardest job you've ever had, but the gains, while slow, will be worth it.
- It's a marathon, not a sprint, so balance is important.
- Progress does not stop after one or two years; keep working if you want more.

CHAPTER 6.

Let Me Talk!

Two years after my stroke, Steve and I attended his graduate school reunion. I had shied away from big social gatherings, but many of my best friends would be there, and I was starting to get more comfortable going out. At one point, conversation turned to charter schools. Opinions flew back and forth on their efficiency, equality, and intent. There was lots of disagreement, but they eventually agreed that larger charter school groups would serve more students more effectively, and funding should be directed that way.

I was silently fuming. Two years earlier, just before my stroke, I had been studying the impact of philanthropy on charter schools. I had met with the principal of a Los Angeles charter school started by community members to serve their low-income, African-American population nearby the kids' homes. It delivered great education on a modest budget and was a pillar of the community. Then the building lease expired, and the community was outbid by a large charter management organization that wanted to start another school to meet their growth goals. The local school had to lease a different building five miles away and bus all their students there.

I had so much I could have shared with this group as they debated a topic I had studied and written about, building expertise as a professor of education! They were coming to conclusions that I thought missed critical aspects of the topic, and yet I couldn't share what I knew with them. I searched for words, racked my brain for ways to hint at the ideas I wanted to contribute. I came up empty. I had much to share and no way to share it. Steve caught my eye, anticipated my growing frustration, and moved us to a new conversation.

. . .

Aphasia is the main communication problem that affects stroke survivors. In *Healing the Broken Brain*, Mike and David Dow explain that aphasia is the "disruption of language," with language referring to the ability to understand what people say to you and say what you mean to others, as well as reading and writing.[41] But the problem differs for each of us. We might understand what others say perfectly but not be able to speak ourselves. Or the other way around. Or some of both. Or have more trouble with reading than listening.

My challenges are primarily expressive: an inability to communicate my thoughts, both speaking and writing. Far more than my limp or lost use of my right arm, substantially diminished speech and writing capability has altered my life the most. It forced me out of teaching; made day-to-day interactions difficult; altered my roles as a mother, wife, and daughter; and made it far harder to build and maintain relationships with others.

Oddly, the language inside my head is not impacted. I still think in words, construct ideas, and even prepare sentences inside my head mostly as before. But when I go to express them externally, I have trouble getting them out, and often the wrong words come out. Steve described my early struggles with aphasia in a CaringBridge entry:

> *Immediately after this last stroke she settled quickly into three reflexive phrases/sentences: 'no, no, no'; 'Is there anything else?' and 'I need a candle.' The first two seem somewhat logical, as thoughts that might have gotten "burned in" just before or during the stroke. The third, no clue . . . It's clear there's a specific thought in her head, but as she concentrates hard on saying it, those are the only words that come. Can't tell you how painful it is to watch her frustration in this.*

If it wasn't so painful, it would almost be funny. Actually, at times it was. "I need a candle" can be a pretty funny response to an unrelated question. Occasionally, even I would crack a smile. But usually I was too focused or too angry to find any humor in the situation. Being able to communicate was more important than ever, and no matter how hard I tried, all that came out were those three damned phrases.

We played endless games of twenty questions that more often than not ended in my even greater fury when they couldn't read my mind after two dozen questions. The confusion was not surprising at all since my thoughts were often disjointed and my responses misleading. Occasionally, after tremendous effort, they would be able to guess what I was trying to say. That was helpful, but it gave me little comfort because my brain was already onto the next unvoiceable thought. For years, every conversation with my family was an opportunity for small improvements since they forced me to correct my sentences when I used the wrong tense, dropped a word, or got lazy. Language is how humans relate to each other, but for me it was another domain of rehab.

· · ·

The National Aphasia Association estimates that about two million people in the United States suffer from aphasia, including about half of all stroke survivors. Even so, it's a little-known condition. The association's 2016 national survey showed that 84.5 percent of the population had never heard of aphasia. Neuroscientist Leora Cherney and her colleagues describe it as "A disturbance of language, resulting from focal damage to the portions of the brain responsible for language, reading, and writing . . . Those affected by aphasia report social isolation, loneliness, loss of autonomy, restricted activities, role changes, and stigmatization."[42]

Aphasia is a loss of language, not a loss of intelligence, but the rest of the world may not see the difference. Strangers might think I am drunk, incompetent, or childish when they first encounter my struggles to communicate. A psychological study titled "The Person with Aphasia and Society" looked at how aphasia can make stroke survivors suddenly feel like outcasts. "Up until the night before the [stroke], the person with aphasia was an integral part of society, considering himself a lifetime member, without questioning his status," wrote the authors.[43] With stroke, and particularly with aphasia, we have reason to doubt our membership in society. Since so much of our identity is constructed through our social relationships, which rely so heavily on language, aphasia can obliterate our feeling of belonging.

Physician Oliver Sacks conveyed this phenomenon brilliantly in his bestseller *The Mind's Eye.* Discussing his patient, Pat, who nearly died from a massive brain hemorrhage and was left completely mute, he wrote:

> *Pat yearned to speak, but was continually frustrated when, after huge efforts to get a word out, it would be the wrong word, or unintelligible. She would try to correct it, but very often would become more unintelligible with every attempt to make herself understood. It started to dawn on her, I think, that her power of speech might never come back, and increasingly she retreated into silence. This inability to communicate was, for her, as for many patients with aphasia, far worse than the paralysis of half her body. I would sometimes see her, in this first year after her stroke, sitting alone in the corridor or in the patients' dayroom, bereft of speech, surrounded by a sort of penumbra of silence, with a stricken and desolate look on her face.[44]*

The fact that I and others with aphasia can still think clearly is a blessing when compared with survivors of many other types of brain trauma. However, this means constant confrontation with our deficit every time we are with others and try to speak. Our normal thought processes are reassuring when we are alone but contribute to intense frustration when we are trying to use them to communicate with others. It's easy to see why survivors with aphasia sometimes withdraw. "When I'm home alone, I don't have aphasia," said a stroke survivor in Barbara Shadden and Joseph Agan's "Renegotiation of Identity."[45]

We are reminded of, and believe in, our old fluency of speech right up until the moment we open our mouths to speak, and then fall short. "The person with aphasia is left with a new identity of communicative incompetence," they wrote. Each time we try to communicate with others, we feel cut off from a world we can no longer participate in.

• • •

The first thing everyone says about Trish Hambridge is that she made them laugh. When her friend and colleague Delia Ansted met her, Trish was playing a practical joke on another coworker at Apple. Delia watched her sneak into a cubicle and quietly remove a set of car keys. Feeling Delia's eyes on her, Trish made a silent shushing gesture before leaving the building and moving the colleague's car. When the coworker returned, convinced her car was stolen, Trish let the panic endure for about ten seconds before revealing the prank and sending the office into a fit of laughter.

"She could go anywhere, be with any group of people, and have a good time. They will all genuinely like her," said Delia. "Some people who just have the kind of personality that strangers respond to. That's Trish." On May 6, 2008, Trish didn't show up for work. Her coworkers and friends worried. They went to her house and knocked down the door, where they found her unconscious on the floor. "I got a call from one of them," remembered Delia, whose own memory of those days is blurry. "She basically said, 'Something bad happened to Trish. She was taken to the emergency room. Nobody knows what it is yet, but I'm headed over there.'"

Trish was forty-three at the time and living alone in California, with her family across the country in New York. She was surrounded by her large group of very close friends. By the time Delia arrived at the hospital, ten other friends were already gathered around Trish, prying information out of the staff until they were kicked out of the emergency room that night. The doctors told them Trish had suffered a "major" ischemic stroke on her left side and had likely been unconscious in her apartment overnight. Delia came back the next day and was one of the first to see Trish.

"She was sitting up and awake and appeared to be alert. But it quickly dawned on me that she really couldn't speak. She was having trouble focusing on what I was saying. She didn't look alarmed. She knew who I was, but she couldn't speak." Like myself, Trish was completely mute immediately after her stroke. She quickly regained her first word, "No." In keeping with her humor, Trish's friends still tease her about that. Since then, she has regained more speech, but she is still severely aphasic.

Like me and many other aphasics, Trish lost her career—she had been a project manager at Apple. Her colleagues and managers were very understanding, but she misses the camaraderie they had in the office on a daily basis. In a relatively short period of time, she saw some of her work friends disappear from her life. She and Delia remain close, but their relationship has had to change, too. Language and stories are such a critical piece of how we bond together; when they go missing, the absence can impact not just the communication, but the relationship itself.

• • •

Like most parts of the stroke experience, aphasia takes on a slightly different form for each survivor. Mike Nickerson, whom I met at a speech therapy program in Chicago, has receptive aphasia. His stroke attacked his posterior left temporal cortex, taking with it his ability to make sense of language, primarily the spoken word. His speech may be grammatically correct, but it is hard to understand because his sentences are peppered with nonexistent or irrelevant words, and he might hear "left" when someone says "right." His struggle with aphasia is less visible than mine, and that can make it even more difficult. In public, he seems to be completely normal, so many people don't understand his hesitations and why he seems lost and confused.

It's different still for Calvin Tashel, who was also at our program in Chicago. When he tries to speak, words don't come out as intended. They are often unrelated to what he was trying to say, and to the listener they seem random and garbled.

Aphasia affects Randy Miller still differently. Since his stroke at age fifty-one, Randy has been unable to hear himself speak, so he doesn't know if the right words are coming out. There is nothing wrong with his hearing; he hears everyone and everything around him just fine. There is simply a disconnect between his speech and the way his brain processes it, so he is always questioning what he's saying. He explained in his halting way, "It's like I can't speak. I can't talk. I can't anything. Speaking is like . . . so close but so far away. I know it's there. It's like right there . . . but now I can't say it, or I can't hear it."

Laure Wang is the most extreme example of lost communication among the survivors I've met. She has locked-in syndrome—unable to move anything but her eyes. She has used several different devices to help her communicate; in various ways, they allow her to speak letter by letter. Early in her recovery, Laure used a DynaVox, which wasn't very user friendly and could take days for just a few sentences. "Many, many a session with DynaVox was spent crying and sweating. I was given a voice, but I hoped for one less frustrating," she said. Laure now uses a spelling board to communicate, most often with a laser pointer, and finds it much easier and less frustrating. It is still far too slow and tedious to convey anything complex or time sensitive, though.

. . .

"When you learn to speak again, it is the most difficult experience that you've ever had," said Sean Maloney. "I used to run an organization with fifteen thousand people, but that's nothing compared to not being able to speak. It's mind-blowing: how do you learn to speak?" Sean was an exceptionally articulate, animated public speaker before his stroke, and having to relearn a skill as fundamental as language was clearly jarring. "It's like going back to childhood. That's incredibly difficult, because 95 percent of people around you don't think you're going to make it." He was frustrated with his aphasia, but even more so, he hated that people would expect, or even think, less of him as soon as they recognized his disability.

In relearning how to speak, both Sean and I spent time learning to "speak with the other side of the brain." The speech center is in the left side of the brain, and music is processed on the right. Melodic Intonation Therapy, a form of therapy that involves singing, takes advantage of this and trains survivors to use tune and rhythm to turn thoughts into lyrics. One year into my recovery, I spent four months in Boston as part of a clinical trial that was rigorously testing the efficacy of this approach; I received ninety minutes of melodic intonation therapy five days a week, and it made a huge difference. While I didn't realize why at the time, my first words at Valley Rehab Hospital had come from singing nursery rhyme songs.

Other experimental therapies, from stem cell implants to intensive speech rehab clinics, can also help. So does more everyday technology: I use Siri's dictation for many text messages or emails, practicing what I want to say and then letting Siri interpret my voice, usually pretty accurately. Trish has become a pro at using tools and apps to help her convey her meaning. She uses an app on her phone called Prologue2Go to help initiate certain words she can't always say right away. She also uses her phone to audibly fill in the blanks in her speech when necessary. For example, Trish might begin a sentence saying, "My dad lives in—" and she'll cue an automated voice that will say, "—Niagara," to complete the sentence. Her dad Doug said, "I don't have a clue how she writes her emails. I know she cuts and pastes, and occasionally she'll get a friend to help her compose it."

Regardless of therapy, apps, or technology, nothing matters as much as continued determination and work. The doctors, therapists, insurance companies, and conventional wisdom that say recovery stops after twelve months are just flat out wrong. My progress feels slow to nonexistent at times, but friends who don't see me often remark how much better my speech is than the last time we spoke. When I think back about where my speech was, I know they are right. I know that progress would not have come without continued therapy, hundreds of Rosetta Stone lessons (Level 1–5 English) on my iPad, and hours on Skype with my mom. Doug said of Trish, "Her determination to get through this and to continue life as best she can is stronger than ever."

Even with continued progress, dealing with aphasia is a constant and frustrating battle that requires adaptation. Making more deliberate choices becomes critical: going to quiet restaurants; small gatherings, not big parties; close friends who can follow your facial expressions rather than strangers who will try (with good intentions) to jump in and complete your sentence for you; and having compassion and patience for yourself. Trish owns her identity as an aphasic stroke survivor, and that choice makes a huge difference. Her friend Delia has seen it work magic. "When waitresses in busy restaurants come over, they're obviously rushed. Trish will say, 'I have a speech problem.' You can feel them calm down, recognizing they're just not going to be able to rush this customer."

• • •

Acclaimed journalist and author Tom Wolfe said of language, "Speech is not one of man's several unique attributes—speech is the attribute of all attributes! Speech is 95 percent plus of what lifts man above animal!"[46] I refuse to accept this. We all use other strategies besides speech to communicate. But it does shed light on just how shattering the challenge of aphasia can be.

Language is humans' most important tool for social participation and community, and it's how we jointly make sense of life and events.[47] Even when we can find ways to work through the challenges or compensate, there's a notable change in what and how we are able to relate to the rest of the world when we lose access to language. Laure's husband Kabir Misra observed, "It takes Laure two minutes to spell out a question, and it interrupts the meeting. It changes the rhythm, and people don't have the time."

In 2017, it was hard to go anywhere without the topic turning to gender dynamics, diversity, and identity. In my academic life, I was considered an expert in those fields. I gave talks, wrote books, and researched these issues. Now, I was mostly confined to passive listening and using vigorous, nonverbal signals to communicate my agreement or disagreement during discussions.

I still hold the knowledge I accumulated before, and I still harbor the same passion that led me to spend years studying these matters. But often, my aphasia prevents me from vocalizing that expertise and passion, from expressing that piece of my identity. "Loss of language equates with some loss of identity as competent social partner and communicator," wrote Barbara Shadden.[48] Without the ability to vocalize what I care about, I can't relate to those around me in the same way, and we derive a huge part of our identity through relationships. We have to find ways to interact and share our values despite our speech deficits.

For years after my stroke, I would not admit in an email that it was written with the help of someone else, even though I clearly could not write on my own. This created confusion and bad expectations. Even after I was no longer denying my stroke, I had not yet come to grips with how to think about myself with reduced access to language. My friend Robin Ely knows that my emails are often cowritten with Steve, and it changed her perception of the message. "I know he's communicating for her. It's her sentiments, she's dictating it, but I know that's just not how Deb would say it," she explained. And she's right. My communication now is no longer mine alone, but a mix of mine and others'. That is true for this book, too. If the thoughts I relay to others are not mine alone, what does that mean for who I am?

. . .

Barbara Shadden has said, "If aphasia came with a warning label, I think it should read, 'Hazardous to identity.'"[49] I agree. At the same time, there are powerful ways we can find to express ourselves through these challenges.

It is often said that 90 percent of daily communication is nonverbal.[50] Whatever the exact number, stroke survivors find creative ways to convey a massive amount through tones and gestures. Just after my stroke, my only word was "no," and I could not even consistently manage a meaningful head shake or nod to answer "yes" or "no" questions. So my family learned to tell "no means no" from "no means yes" by my tone and by watching my eyes to see if I looked surprised or frustrated that I had just said "no" when my head meant "yes." This wasn't perfectly accurate, but it was a start. Before long, we were using our own version of twenty questions and my various versions of "no" to arrive at more and more thoughts.

Oliver Sacks' patient, Pat, also found ways to communicate nonverbally:

> *She began to discover that she could communicate in ways*
> *that didn't require speech. She had developed a knack for*
> *understanding other people by their gestures and expressions as*
> *much as their words. She could indicate her own thoughts and*

*feelings not by speech, but by eloquent gesture and mime . . . she
regained her ability to communicate, albeit differently, she was
able to regain a life that reflected what was most important to
her before her stroke. "'Nothing has changed since her stroke,' her
daughter said. 'She has all her old loves and passions' . . . [51]*

Trish also chose to go back out into the world and re-create her social
identity. Always quick-witted, Trish misses the fact that she can't crack
jokes quite like she used to, but she doesn't let it steal her fire. She's just as
hilarious with the tools she has at hand. Her expressive tone of voice often
conveys even more than words ever could, and with a few programmed
sentences on her iPhone app.

Even without speech, Trish can still throw out a punchline right on
cue and crack up a room full of people. She finds new ways to bring out her
personality now that her speech is impaired. As she told me in our interview,
"Hilarious is me."

LET ME TALK!: CHAPTER 6 HIGHLIGHTS

- Aphasia, a set of disabilities affecting communication, can take many forms; it affects stroke survivors in very different ways and to various degrees, from severe to not at all.

- Speech and language impact nearly every part of life and are a key way we not only communicate but relate to other people.

- The right speech therapy can continue to reverse the impact of aphasia for years.

- We can learn to communicate more nonverbally and use other tools.

- Building your own strategies to deal with aphasia is very important.

CHAPTER 7.

Grief

October 9, 1995, had been a good day. My mother had taken a quick flight from Los Angeles to get her baby fix and had spent the day with three-month-old Sarah and her two older brothers—almost four and six at the time. I dropped her at the airport, returned to kiss the already sleeping kids, and drifted off to sleep with Steve. I woke up a few hours later to a call from my brother. When mom got home, she found my father drowned in their backyard pool. He was just sixty-four at the time, completely healthy. Now, in an instant, he was gone. I was in shock. I spent six hours shaking with tears, and much of the next several years on the border of depression (something I did not realize until many years later). I still miss my dad dearly, but thanks to family, counseling, a great support network, and time, I moved past the intense grief that accompanied that sudden and devastating loss.

June 4, 2013, eighteen years later, was not a good day. Three years after my stroke, I had reached the end of the allowable medical leave at Stanford. Steve and I had a meeting with Claude Steele, then dean of the Stanford Education School. With great compassion, he explained that since I had not regained enough speech to fulfill my role as a professor, I would have to give up my tenured position at Stanford.

I was devastated. When I got home, I cried; I stared into space; I punched pillows; I collapsed into Steve's arms. Repeat. For three years, I had worked so hard to recover, rebuild, and reclaim my old self. I had failed! The emotions I felt that day were reminiscent of the night I lost my dad. It wasn't just my position and profession that I had lost: that day, I was forced to face head-on the fact that my old self had been taken away from me. Without realizing it at the time, I was grieving the loss of my own identity.

. . .

Nearly every survivor I talked to spoke of some level of depression in their journey. Clinical depression affects one out of three stroke survivors, and it often goes undiagnosed. Depression can be triggered by the physical damage to the brain as well as by the emotional trauma. Biochemical changes in the brain that result from stroke can increase the likelihood of depression. For example, if cell death occurs in a certain region of the brain, the survivor may not be able to feel positive emotions, explains Dr. Robert Robinson, a psychiatrist at the University of Iowa who studies poststroke depression. "All the tips, tricks, reframings, and forced optimism in the world may not be able to overcome a new biological disposition in which professional help and likely medication would be recommended."[52] This impact is often underappreciated, and thus, psychological support is usually minimal or nonexistent as survivors and health-care pros focus on physical recovery.

Some counselors and therapists, witnessing the experiences of patients like me after I lost my tenure, compare the experience of stroke to bereavement. Many draw on the stages of grief model in their work to help stroke survivors. This road map for the grieving process was drawn up by Elisabeth Kübler-Ross in her 1969 book, *On Death and Dying*.[53] Dr. Kübler-Ross suggested that grief was a process that embraced five stages: denial, anger, bargaining, depression, and acceptance (not necessarily in linear order).

"I think the Kübler-Ross model is an invaluable tool for helping patients gain perspective on what they're going through—their emotional journey—and to realize they are not alone in their experience," said neuropsychologist

Monique Tremaine, director of psychology and neuropsychology services at Kessler Institute of Rehabilitation in West Orange, New Jersey. Since my stroke, I have felt each of these to some degree, and others do as well. "Survivors readily identify with the stages and can accept the fact that they will move forward and backward through them with changing levels of recovery and life circumstances."[54]

This model also suggests ways to cope with the depression that can accompany stroke: striving for some degree of acceptance. Rather than constantly looking back at our old selves, we must learn to look forward. Small wins, conscious choices, and finding new ways to live a meaningful life can help bring us out of the backward-facing grasp of grief. It's not always possible, and not so clear-cut. Denial can help motivate hard work early after a stroke, and that would help survivors regain more functionality. "Striking a balance between reality and hope can be difficult, and acceptance should be discussed in terms of the here and now," said Dr. Tremaine.

Finding the right ways to anticipate, acknowledge, and move past the grief can be critical to unlocking a happy poststroke life. Lisa Levine-Sporer spoke about Sean Maloney's journey as less a pure loss and more a rebirth: "I also think that some stroke survivors go through a loss, as if there was a death," she said. "It's just an acknowledgment of a different identity."

. . .

I met Malik Thoma at a therapy clinic, where we bonded over our furious determination to regain the use of our affected hands. His stroke impacted the right side of his brain, so he does not suffer from aphasia and can share his story more freely. The son of Indian immigrants and raised Muslim, Malik had begun to live out the American dream. He was founder and CEO of a chain of day spas with more than ninety employees, and he had plans to expand his operation and acquire eleven more.

Malik also felt an immense sense of pride in his work, since his spas trained and hired battered women, giving them stable jobs in a location away from their abusers. Malik had created his business out of a passion: his intention was to provide jobs to the women that needed them most. Using proceeds from the company, he would team up with shelters and pay for training for women who were ready to go into the workforce, then he would guarantee a job for them at one of his facilities when they graduated.

Big things were happening with the business, but the hours were grueling, and the pace frenetic. "I was always putting out little fires, doing long-range planning, putting in new systems," he said. His second son had just been born, and he and his family were planning to move from Arizona to California.

Malik was actually on his way to the doctor to get a blood test when he got a call about a homeless man whom he had previously befriended. Wanting to help him out of a jam, he went to see him and paid for the man to get his car fixed. And then he went to Costco to buy the man a one-year membership to 24-Hour Fitness so he could use their showers and facilities.

During that detour, he suffered his stroke. Malik said regretfully, "Had I gone to my doctor's appointment, none of this would have happened. I feel like I was betrayed by God." Of all the survivors I've met, Malik has had perhaps the hardest emotional journey. He has almost entirely lost his faith. His relationship with his wife, which was already strained, deteriorated further as a result of the stresses of the stroke and recovery process. Malik tried going back to running his company, but the stroke left him with double vision that made it incredibly difficult. This lack of professional productivity has shattered his self-image, and he believes that he is a poor role model for his kids. He is unable to do many of the activities he did prior to the stroke, impacting his health and physique.

After selling his chain of day spas and wanting to feel productive again, Malik labored long and hard over an application to join the board of trustees of a local community college. What once would have taken a few hours was now a two-day process that left him mentally exhausted, drained by the double vision that hampers every task. After all the hard work, he did not get the position. "I wanted to give, but I'm not even accepted for those positions . . . I have all of these grandiose plans to help humanity, and now I can't even help myself."

Malik is in an incredibly difficult situation that would discourage even the most optimistic among us. Yet his continued negativity and pessimism even years after his stroke are at least partially self-fulfilling. "Nothing physical is available to me," he told me. He walks with a limp but is not constrained to a wheelchair. His exercise of choice may no longer be available, but there are physical activities that he could do with some persistence and creativity.

Malik has thought about ending it all: twice he has put a gun in his mouth, the trigger cocked. His situation has been made even harder by a fractured family. His wife has told him on multiple occasions that he has "ruined her life." Optimism in the face of these circumstances is extremely hard, maybe even irrational. But if he attempted to reframe the narrative, that could lead to a healthier outlook and a happier poststroke life.

· · ·

This feeling of grief that Malik experiences is not uncommon among people who have suffered medical trauma. "When ill persons attempt to return to the normal world and fail, they usually feel profound disappointment and grief for their lost self-images," writes Professor Kathy Charmaz. As failures and disappointments add up, they can begin to see the feeling as permanent and themselves as a burden, becoming passive and isolated rather than attempting to shape their own life more actively. In short, "they accept a discredited self."[55]

Malik's failed attempts to go back to work or to an honorary position left him distraught, convinced that he couldn't take care of himself, let alone help those around him. In trying to live his previous life, he felt deficits in every level of Maslow's pyramid: basic function, belonging to his old communities, and achievement in his old domain. "I have accomplished nothing in the last four and a half years," he lamented—a statement that is only accurate when measured against the yardstick of his former life.

It was very hard to get Malik to talk about the future. He didn't see any way toward a life of meaning. He returned frequently to his anger—at his sister who intervened, at his wife who didn't support him the way he thought she could have, and at his mother who often took charge in ways that he sometimes thought did more harm than good. Contrast that with Laure Wang, who has locked-in syndrome, cannot move below the neck, and has to use a speech board to talk with her eyes. Yet she has used the stroke to redefine who she is and finds herself able to live a rewarding life.

Survivors adapt more successfully if they can proactively recognize when they fall into a chaos narrative and try to position themselves differently—to seek rebuilding and growth given the new situation, rather than comparing their current life with their old one. Many survivors have taken steps to focus themselves on building meaningful connections in new communities and enhancing esteem in new ways. Of course, this is not easy and requires a willingness to accept and seek support.

• • •

After my stroke, I was constantly anxious about my speech progress. My therapist recognized early on that I had "performance anxiety" and prescribed a small dose of antidepression medications that helped immensely. In *The Happiness Hypothesis*, psychologist Jonathan Haidt explores the critical factors that lead to a happy life.[56] He named one of them the cortical lottery: certain chemical patterns in the brain predict a happier disposition. He thinks SSRIs (a class of antidepressants) are a great solution when appropriate.

With so much focus on physical disabilities and recovery, stroke survivors often do not get the emotional resources they need. After my father died, I was encouraged to seek therapy (and thankfully had insurance that covered it). Though a stroke can be an even more traumatic experience, the grief and damage to personal identity after stroke has not been articulated or understood by society in a way that encourages therapy. Doctors rarely recommend or prescribe it. Studies show that many patients who do have depression after stroke do not receive treatment for it, said Dr. Robinson.

Given the physical and emotional trauma, as well as the biological impact of stroke, psychological support should be more forthcoming. Unfortunately, it's not often part of standard treatment. Many doctors as well as family members tend to explain away depression as an understandable response to the loss and impairment that stroke produces.[57]

I met Melanie Drane, a psychotherapist based in Los Angeles, at the Rehabilitation Institute of Chicago. I was participating in an intensive aphasia program and she was there to support a close friend who was there, as well. Melanie's sister had passed away from a stroke, and since then, she has devoted a portion of her counseling career to helping stroke survivors with aphasia and advocating for resources in the stroke world. "It is a battle to get stroke survivors to come through the door. Many are suffering silently and don't necessarily think of seeking helpful resources. Others simply don't have access to resources," she said.

Of course, those who do seek support often cannot get it. "Even in a city like Los Angeles, there is virtually no one out there," said Drane, referring to counselors with specialized knowledge about stroke survivors, especially those with aphasia. Plus, most stroke survivors have to fight for bare-minimum treatment and rehab. For so many survivors who decide to confront the emotional challenges and manage to find qualified support, the cost of counseling services is unthinkable. Lack of psychological support resources are another way that socioeconomic position may play a dramatic role in recovery. Given the lack of attention paid to the need for therapy, those without substantial means typically do not see a professional psychologist for help, or they choose to dedicate finite resources toward more tangible recovery efforts such as physical, speech, or occupational therapy, some of which insurance may partially cover.

Other avenues can help the battle with grief, as well. I've picked up meditation, which has helped me keep calm and reset my frame of mind when needed. For some, turning to faith has been critical for this part of recovery. In fact, my neurologist Dr. Chitra Venkatasubramanian (Venkat) thinks that faith plays a role in how different populations bounce back from stroke. "Ninety-five percent of the African-American families that I've had as my patients are very faith based. For them, church provides enormous support. For them, it's God. It's God's will, and God will show us a miracle, or God will take care of it. This faith in God is huge for them," she said.

Drawing on deeper values like this can help some survivors not just get through the grief but also grow from it. "At first I was sad, filled with self-pity and depression," said Laure Wang. "But because of my faith, I made it through my suffering by becoming stronger and better . . . God has made me a better person, and the old angst and fear have gone away. I like the new me more." This deeper meaning can also be found in a renewed desire to help others (like other stroke survivors) or to play a stronger role in their kids' lives.

Until recently, psychologists had always considered two possible outcomes with trauma victims: some struggled with depression and perhaps developed PTSD; others showed resilience and bounced back. There is a third path, and when Adam Grant shared it with Sheryl Sandberg, she didn't believe it. "Post-traumatic growth? Too catch-phrasy. Too unlikely," she said. However, she grew to believe in it and wrote a book describing it. Her intro to *Option B* ends with a perfect line to describe how I feel about battling back from stroke: "Life is never perfect. We all live some form of Option B. This book is to help us all kick the shit out of it."[58]

GRIEF: CHAPTER 7 HIGHLIGHTS

- Grief is normal, and some depression, too; after all, life as we knew it, and some elements of our identity, have been taken away.
- Survivors who suffer from clinical depression should consult with a professional.
- There is not nearly enough recognition of the emotional challenges for stroke survivors and their families, or resources to support them. Ask for it.
- We should all seek emotional help and support, in various forms.
- Post-traumatic growth really is possible with the right attitude and support.

CHAPTER 8.

Lean On

For the first few months after my stroke, Steve would post regular updates about my progress on CaringBridge. These posts triggered many supportive comments from my friends and family. I was not aware of these messages for a while, but on October 24, he wrote to our community:

> *I'm now regularly reading posts to Deb (as well as cards and letters). I can tell she can't stand that all these people are worrying about her (surprised?!) AND that she is extremely touched and appreciative. So thanks again . . . and do keep the positive energy flowing whenever and however you choose to do so.*

I've never been one to look for compliments. In fact, I am criticized for my inability to take them. However, I loved having Steve read me the outpouring of support while I lay in my hospital bed. They reaffirmed my determination and enthusiasm to fight this thing with every ounce of strength and grit I had.

Our good friend Monique Johnson, whose sons are close to my boys, wrote, "Please know that we are with you in spirit and stand by ready to offer support—from a simple text, to a hug, to anything at all. We've no doubt that no one is better suited to overcoming this challenge than you, Deb, and that you are surrounded by an amazing family who will help get you through the toughest moments." Comments like this had a powerful effect on me. Though it would take time and introspection for me to fully embrace the available support, they showed me that I had friends and family surrounding me who were eager to help in any way they could. My emotions may have been dominated by anger and fear, but the outpouring of support let me also feel gratitude for such an incredibly powerful network to lean on.

A support network's role goes far beyond comfort in the immediate aftermath of stroke. For me, family, friends, caregivers, organizations like PSA, and the inspirational stories of survivors captured in this book haven't just been motivating, they have been essential to helping me rediscover my values and rebuild my life over the past eight years. My life is what it is today because of those around me.

. . .

Even without trauma, our social networks play a critical role in our lives. Studies consistently find a positive link between our social support and psychological well-being, including physical health.[39] So it makes sense that researchers and doctors have found that a strong support network is absolutely necessary to stroke recovery. "It increasingly seems to me that [strong bonds of family and social connections] is not just a bonus but essential," says Dr. Venkat. "That's something we've seen over and over again."

We are all inclined to turn to friends and family in the face of traumatic events. Hope and motivation are certainly one way they help and can inspire us to work hard on recovery. But the long, taxing physical and emotional recovery after stroke is different from grieving a death or other events that rally our supporters. Such networks play a significant role not just in mental well-being but also in the actual physical recovery. "The person who has a great social support system will go farther, will adapt to what's going on, and will be able to achieve more in terms of stroke recovery," said Dr. Venkat. "It's these intangible, unmeasurable factors that also go a long way toward improving outcomes; no question about it."

Having friends and family who can help with minor concerns allows us to focus more fully on the big jobs. My family jokes that, "Mom had a stroke, and we got fat," because of the influx of meals our friends delivered when I was in the hospital and beyond. One of our closest friends, Kim Menninger, quickly organized a food brigade, with dozens of friends dropping precooked meals in our garage fridge immediately after my stroke and many coordinating to continue deliveries for months after. Support like this not only enabled me to focus single-mindedly on my recovery, but allowed my family to focus more of their time and energy on helping me and each other.

A strong support network also plays a more subtle role: it helps to reestablish our newly challenged identity, giving clarity, direction, and priority to the recovery process. In many cases, stroke recovery is a long journey with constant frustrations and many mountains to climb. It is easy to feel isolated and overwhelmed. With those we love around us, we have a reminder of what we share and value in common. Our support network helps us focus on what matters, envision what we want to achieve, and motivate us to pursue it.

· · ·

Kathy Howard was fifty-five years old, an office manager for an outpatient treatment program, struggling to get her two children through college. She typically came home from work exhausted, so she was inactive and overweight. When she was rushed to the hospital in the wake of her stroke, the doctors asked how long she had been diabetic. "I don't have diabetes," she told them. She was wrong. Her stroke was a wake-up call. With support, her recovery has included a full lifestyle change.

Not long after her stroke, Kathy was supposed to attend a high school reunion the day before a planned stroke-awareness walk. Feeling self-conscious about her poststroke disabilities, she tried to back out of the reunion. "I didn't want anybody to see me walking funny." she said. "But I have this one friend I have known since I was five, and she said, 'You are not missing this.' We went . . . and I was scared to death. What if I can't get there? What if I can't find a bathroom? What if this or that?"

In the end, she had such a great time at the reunion and felt so much support that she decided to send an email to see if anybody wanted to attend the stroke-awareness walk with her. "I went to a small school, but about twenty girls showed up." The next walk she organized had high school friends, doctors, nurses, and family—sixty-five people came to support her and stroke awareness.

Kathy still has regular pain, and in her left side she feels a buzzing or burning sensation. "On days when it's really bad, it's like somebody is scraping cut glass or sticking tacks or sandpaper on my face." Yet, she still views the stroke, at least in part, as a blessing. Her husband Jim has been a rock of support, filling her journey with good spirit and humor. And he credits her broad network for more of the same, "Because of the person she is, she had tons of support." Just as they persuaded her not to back out of her reunion, her friends have been instrumental in providing a supportive and encouraging environment. "I'm blessed with a lot of girlfriends, and that is huge," she said.

• • •

Support may be critical, but it isn't always easy to accept, even when generously and genuinely offered. In my past life, I was an independent, determined (some would say stubborn) woman. Rarely did I need or want my husband's help or help from my colleagues. So, embracing new supports and constraints did not come naturally to me. Steve's CaringBridge update on October 30, almost two months after my stroke, was a fairly typical story of my early days:

*I arrived at the hospital to find Deb absolutely furious with
the nurses. Lots of "no, no, no" in an angry voice, pushing them
away, and fist waving behind their backs. They had found her in
the bathroom in the wheelchair. She had transferred herself from
bed to chair—an absolute no no— and they were understandably
upset with her.*

I did learn to observe some hospital rules over time. I found that while I
battled to reclaim some independence, ironically, I had to accept support at
times. My family had to trust that I would ask for help when needed and not
overdo it. Only then would they trust me enough to leave me alone without
worrying about more rebellious acts like my wheelchair escape. In time, I
could climb stairs on my own, get dressed on my own, and later drive on my
own. But I had to build up to these accomplishments, accepting that I didn't
and likely never would have the independence I had before.

As I've recalibrated, the meaning of independence has also changed for
me. It's critically important that I can survive on my own and be my own
person. But where I used to yell, "Let me talk," at the first hint of help,
frustrated with others' impatience and desperate to communicate, I now look
more often to Steve or my kids to help communicate when that can be clearer
or more efficient. It's not so important that I be seen as someone who never
needs help. In fact, it makes me wonder why I had always been afraid about
seeking help before. I used to be so afraid of that particular vulnerability.

Of course, with disability we are dependent on others to a greater degree
than we'd like—from small things like putting in contact lenses to massive
tasks like needing cowriters and collaborators to write this book. Feelings of
embarrassment and incompetence, and fears of being a burden, have all been part
of my poststroke state of mind. Other survivors have had the same experience. In
one study, Charmaz found that chronically ill people tend to lead a restricted life,
be socially isolated, feel discredited, and feel they are a burden to others.

Once I opened up and overcame my fears, I saw how ready and willing to help those around me were, and I could accept their support. I also started to see a life among a strong support network could be not only tolerable but preferable. Early in my planning for this book, I traveled to Minnesota to attend the annual meeting of a small group of organizational behavior faculty and graduate students from around the country. These get-togethers had been happening regularly for about nine years at that time (and they continue today), and we called them the "May Meaning Meetings," organized by Professor Amy Wrzesniewski. Like many high-pressure professional jobs, at times academia can feel like a rat race. In order to get tenure at most universities, you have to publish a lot of articles or books. A group of academics from around the country convenes each year to step away and ask ourselves how we could stay focused on making a difference through our work. How, in the face of the professional pressure, could we support each other to accomplish work that we personally found meaningful? The gatherings are small, usually about thirty people, so the conversations can be more personal and go a little deeper than what happens in larger groups. Rather than projecting strength and confidence as we did all year, we welcomed the opportunity to open up, question ourselves, and be supported.

Beyond my limited engagements back at Stanford, the 2014 May Meaning Meeting was the first academic event I chose to attend after my stroke. My struggle to find meaning was particularly relevant at that point, and this was the safest space I could find in my professional domain. Like everyone else there, I had the opportunity to give a twenty-minute talk in two smaller sessions of about ten people each. It was just a few months after I had given my "Lucky to Be Alive" presentation at a Pacific Stroke Association conference. I used much of that presentation again, but this time I added a section about my idea for this book, incorporating some feedback I'd gotten from my support group, longtime friends Amy Beringer, Patty Collier, Lisa Kelley, Patty Jackson, Ann Mathieson, Sue Panella, Su-Moon Paik, and Nancy Ryan.

The May Meaning Meeting delivered on its name. The group rallied around my ideas, pushed me to think more deeply about my experience and how I could use it to help others, and helped me commit to the book project. They didn't just motivate me—they helped me identify one way I could find meaning in my poststroke reality.

• • •

Unfortunately, much-needed support can be elusive for some survivors. Mary Jones lived in the Washington, DC, area before her stroke. She relished being surrounded by history, culture, and nature. She took day trips to the mountains and the beach and spent long afternoons at museums on the National Mall. Two of her favorite pastimes were golf and going on walks with her two bichon frise dogs.

On September 11, 2006, Mary was struck by a headache as she prepared for a fundraising event she was coordinating for the local animal rescue shelter. She doesn't remember much of what happened, but she believes the stroke was quickly diagnosed upon her arrival at the hospital. Initially unable to walk, Mary was confined to a wheelchair with paralysis on the entire left side of her body. Her memory function took a hit, and she became blind in her left eye, so is unable to drive. After extensive therapy and a lot of practice walking, Mary has regained some of her mobility, but she still only has functionality in one arm. Cooking is very tough, so her diet suffered. Mary's health crisis kicked off a downward spiral of events. She was bedridden and had to wear diapers for incontinence. That, and all the other support she needed put quite a strain on her husband, who was her primary caregiver for three years.

One day, quite out of the blue, Mary's husband called her family in her hometown of St. Louis to tell them, "I'm done with this. I'm packing up all Mary's stuff, and I'm sending her to St. Louis, and I'm filing for

divorce. You guys can take care of her." And that's what happened. Mary
loved her life on the East Coast, still had hopes of being able to return to
her old job at some point, and never wished to go back to St. Louis. But
she had no choice.

Mary was forty-four when her family placed her in a retirement home,
where she spent three full years surrounded by senior citizens, some twice
her age. Rather than getting the support she needs, she's been taken
advantage of: family members and caregivers have both stolen from her.

• • •

Unfortunately, Mary's situation is not unique, particularly in the United
States. Our culture can isolate us from family and values independence, so
we are less inclined to care for each other. "We have more nursing homes
here than in the whole world put together," said therapist and educator
Waleed Al-Oboudi. Just when people need support the most, they get
pushed out into a place where they live even more alone. Many stroke
survivors acutely feel this absence of support. A literature review conducted
by Murray, Young, Forster, and Ashworth revealed that the most common
long-term problem identified by stroke patients and their carers was lack of
emotional support.[60]

"It was just so scary and so big, and I felt so alone," said Andrea Helft.
"You're the only person going through it, really . . . It is too bad I didn't
have peers to talk to. That would have been really great." She said that is the
one thing she would change—having therapy or support for the emotional
component of the journey. In the end, Andrea was able to find ways to feel
supported and "hang her hat on some progress." But it wasn't easy. She's
an extreme extrovert: "Almost all of my good feelings come from being
with other people," she said. She looked for "anything to not feel so alone."
Of course, when dealing with the physical limitations imposed by stroke,

everything is harder. "I tried to go online and find people, but I couldn't see. I couldn't read the computer to do that kind of search."

Despite the consensus that emotional support is critical to recovery and that many people in our society lack it, there are shockingly few resources available. Insurance covers physical, speech, and occupational therapy (though often way too little), but usually no emotional therapies. Survivors are not systematically encouraged to seek out support groups, and families have little access to networks that provide training or resources to help them support the stroke survivor. Without that, we lose the chance to learn from all those who have gone through this before us and to make the journey a team effort rather than a solo mission.

• • •

Often, even those who seek to support stroke survivors—or anybody going through a hard time—simply don't know how. I do not blame those who struggle with this. I remember myself fumbling when a friend was most in need. "I'm sorry," or "I don't know what to say," or "Are you OK?" come out as inadequate tropes.

Being on the receiving side, effective support makes a big difference. Eight years into my recovery, I draw on my support network deeply and often. Many of the reservations I had about doing so have faded, and the value is clearer than ever. Yet I still find times when I'm reluctant to reach out to certain people who I know care deeply and have been critical supporters in the past because they simply don't help much. Having now gone through this process and learned from others, I have a better understanding of what makes support effective.

Immediately after my stroke, I avoided most social interactions, so even some close friends didn't see me for a while. When they did, most were loving and supportive and treated me as an old friend. Many offered a small, frustrating, but appreciated "You look like you're doing great." But some, either out of discomfort or an intentional desire to not treat me as just a stroke survivor, didn't even acknowledge the situation. This is isolating. "The two things we want to know when we're in pain are that we're not crazy to feel the way we do and that we have support. Acting like nothing significant is happening to people in need denies us that," wrote Sandberg and Grant in *Option B*.[61]

Perhaps the most important thing I've learned is that it's important to acknowledge the situation and need but not make the interaction completely about it. Recovering from stroke certainly changes my needs and dominates my concerns, but stroke survivor is only one part of my identity. I am a person beyond that, and the best supporters can acknowledge and give attention to both at the same time.

Sandberg wrote about the difference it made when a colleague asked, "How are you doing *today*?" The addition implies that the person isn't looking for a general update on state of mind but rather is acknowledging that every day is a different challenge and that he or she is seeking to help in the moment. This becomes natural to those closest to the situation who see all the ups and downs, but it may take more thoughtfulness for those who aren't so close.

When Steve was planning for my return home after two months in various hospitals, Kevin Menninger, a good family friend and structural engineer by day, confirmed with Steve that I'd need a left-side handrail going both up and down the stairs to our second- floor bedroom, and told him that unless Steve said otherwise, he'd just install it. This was a great example of finding ways to help, a far deeper form of support than expressing a desire to. As Sandberg also wrote, asking someone, "What can I do to help?" can actually add to the person's burden when you are trying to do the opposite. Suggesting even a small way to be helpful both shows thoughtful support and saves them the energy and discomfort of making a response and finding things to ask for.

Karen Jordan, an immensely thoughtful friend who has become much closer in the past eight years, sent Steve an email shortly after my stroke. "I know you and Deb used to run with Kaya (our dog), and I'm guessing she's not getting much exercise these days. Unless you tell me otherwise, I'll swing by the house and take her walking with my dogs when we go out, starting tomorrow." It may seem like a tiny thing, but it showed a deep and thoughtful desire to be truly helpful during a hard time—and it was. Steve didn't even know he was stressing about that, and never would have thought to ask someone for help. But when Karen made the offer, he felt a deep sense of appreciation.

· · ·

After the rally of support around the initial trauma, it's unfortunately common for networks to fade over time. Only dedicated networks are willing to stick around for the years or lifetime of required support. "Both stroke survivors and their families note that pre-stroke social networks seem to dissolve, leaving them with a restricted support network of family and sometimes close friends," found a study of stroke's impact on identity.[62]

Psychologist Susan Silk devised the ring theory for trauma supporters. *Option B* describes it well: "She suggests writing down the names of people in the center of the tragedy and then drawing a circle around them. Next draw a bigger circle around that one and write the names of the people who are the next most affected by the loss . . . "[63] And so on. In our case, I was in the middle, Steve in the next ring, then my mom and our kids, and so on. "Wherever you are in the circle, offer comfort in and seek comfort out," they suggest. This structure ensures a sustainable support system that won't burn out with time.

Some communities and religious organizations provide this kind of extended support more naturally. Dr. Venkat describes patterns she has seen:

I've had patients say, "If only I can just go back to church and read the Bible and be part of this group." For them, that's a key aspect of support.

I don't think I have ever seen an Asian trauma survivor without family support. I just have not seen it.

[On African-American families] They fall into two groups. One has really good family support—if grandma's sick, the grandson's there. The grandson advocates for grandma and makes sure she gets to all the appointments. He's drops everything and drives grandma wherever she needs to go, and he's there for all the therapy sessions. This group usually lives together in the same household or very close. With the other group, there's no family support at all. There's no middle ground between the two.

Different cultures will always have different family norms and dynamics, and I wonder if, in our western world, individuals have become too isolated. We value independence and individual freedoms more than ever, and strong nuclear families are still typical (though even that is shifting). But our communities and ties beyond that are far weaker than they used to be. Religion is on the decline and community centers are out of vogue. Large families and tribes, the norm in human history, were built to endure traumas as a group. Our modern society has lost that emphasis. My mother was extremely close to her large extended family, but my kids barely know theirs.

• • •

When support isn't strong enough, sometimes stroke survivors must take matters into their own hands. After three years in the retirement home in St. Louis, Mary woke up one morning and thought, "The only thing they do for me here is provide meals." It would be difficult, but she could prepare meals for herself. So, she moved out of the retirement home and into her own apartment. She found a church in St. Louis and built some good relationships there. She has made a good friend, also called Mary, who is a fellow stroke survivor. They meet at the mall a few times each week to have lunch and hang out. "My quality of life just shot through the roof. It's much better." This has allowed her to reclaim more independence and more of the benefits of a support network.

These networks provide far more than meals and medical care. The members care and are cared for, nourishing not just physiological but psychological needs as well. Mary now chooses whom she spends time with and is around others who want to spend time with her. The circumstances and people are different, but the general need for social encouragement and connection is the same. And she has found it.

Mary has moved up to higher needs in Maslow's pyramid. The lower requirements of food, safety, and security may be a bit tougher than at the retirement home, but she can still meet them. Now she can build a true sense of belonging in a community she chooses to be a part of, and she has the freedom to build a new life that is more meaningful and fulfilling.

Kathy Howard, blessed with a great support network herself, recognized the importance of support resources, and that for many, there just weren't enough of them. She took it on herself to help fill that gap. "I visit a lot of new survivors. It's my passion. I love being able to walk into a room and say, 'You know, I was one of those people who was told I might not ever walk again, but I drove over here to see you.'" She said the connection with someone who has been there is huge. And it provides strong motivation when survivors meet someone who has not just reclaimed physical abilities but also has independence and mental happiness.

Thankfully, my family was blessed with strong outer rings of friends who have acted like family. When Steve wrote in CaringBridge that I was contemplating a move to Boston for melodic intonation therapy, Robin Ely immediately emailed Steve to say their spare room was mine if I wanted it. She and her family gave me both support and independence, and a true home away from home. At home, our friends supported me in every way and, nearly as important, supported my family as they supported me.

LEAN ON: CHAPTER 8 HIGHLIGHTS

- Support networks are critical for people in hard times–ask for help.
- Stroke recovery can be harder to support effectively than other traumas, as the journey is both uncertain and long-lasting.
- Supporters need support, too–encourage those in the "outer rings" of your support network to help anyone who is closer in.
- Many people mean well but just aren't sure how to provide support. When interacting, try to acknowledge a survivor's full identity, not just their trauma; and be proactive in finding specific ways to be helpful, not just offering to help.

CHAPTER 9.

Stroke Is a Family Illness

Two years after my stroke, my daughter Sarah was giving a talk at her
school to four hundred students, teachers, and parents. The weekly
"Chapel Talk" was a tradition for the high school seniors. Steve and I were
in attendance, and Sarah hadn't shared anything with us beforehand. So we
listened anxiously with everyone else to her story:

-----

*September 3, 2010: I'm a very excited high school sophomore
stoked for the long weekend ahead.*

*September 5, 2010: I'm a terrified teenager watching her life
change forever.*

-----

*Imagine spending eight helpless, clueless hours alone with your
dog, stuck in a condo, while your role model and mom is carted from
Truckee Hospital to Reno Hospital. You have no information other
than a harried phone call from your oldest brother and dad telling
you, "We think Mom is having a stroke."*

Imagine getting pulled over for speeding on the way to the hospital.

*Imagine the strongest, most independent, most stubborn, and
most influential person in your life; imagine her struggling to tell the
nurse that her speech is fine when asked to form a complete sentence.*

*Imagine a grueling, five-hour drive getting you home at
5:00 a.m. while your dad and continuously deteriorating mom are
airlifted to Stanford.*

Imagine going to the hospital after a few sleepless hours, spent imagining the worst and being told you can't even go into the emergency room because you aren't sixteen yet.

Imagine, after jumping through all imaginable hoops, being allowed to see your mom. Imagine the worst; imagine seeing your mom completely paralyzed on her right side and unable to make a sound or express herself in any way.

Now imagine going to school the next day and trying to pretend that nothing had happened. I've always been private and independent; I always thought I was so strong. These last two years can be described in countless ways, but I prefer to see them as a journey into what it truly means to be strong.

September 7, 2010: I went to school as I did every morning, pretending I had the same fun-filled Labor Day that all of my friends had. Nobody knew of my mom's stroke except my best friend who was in Tahoe with me that weekend, and even she didn't know the severity.

My dad had sent emails to all of my teachers informing them of my situation, but I refused any help and extensions offered. When [Mr.] McWright asked to see me so he could check in, I thought it was a waste of time.

If I fell behind, let my grades slip, or asked for any help beyond the usual, I was weak. I couldn't be weak. If I was weak, I let my family down.

And yet, for that first week when none of my friends knew the truth, every laugh was a stab of guilt and every tear a source of shame.

I went to school, kept up my grades, and went to Stanford Hospital after school to visit mom and do homework.

Gradually, I started telling my friends, one at a time, what had happened. They were incredible. They offered me rides home and places to work away from the chaos.

My support network was a net ready to catch me if I fell. My friends' families were among the many that made dinner for us in the months following the stroke; catching rides home with friends became routine.

Come to think of it, getting those rides were probably the first times I had asked anyone for help after mom's stroke.

To put the chaos of my family's poststroke life in perspective, our situation was not that of the average poststroke family.

For anyone who doesn't know, when a person has a stroke, they're kept in the ICU so doctors can make sure they're stable before getting them out to therapy. The faster a stroke patient starts therapy, the more effective the therapy is.

My mom wasn't in the ICU for the typical three days—she couldn't leave. The doctors had no freaking clue what had caused the stroke. To give you an idea of how weird her situation was, I should tell you that every Monday, Stanford hospital does a case study where they bring in the heads of any major departments connected to the case and a whole bunch of med students and just try and figure out what's going on.

My mom was that case study not once but three times, which means that she was in the ICU for three weeks.

During those three weeks, I was commuting to the hospital almost every day after soccer practice. I was terrified, stressed, and, most importantly, closed down. My friends knew my mom had had a severe stroke, but that was all they knew.

I didn't really understand the medical technicalities then. So, if I had tried to explain what had happened in detail to friends, they couldn't have fully appreciated the severity of the situation. I didn't even try to tell them. I was a big girl; why should people know I was scared? I could handle it on my own.

After three weeks, my mom was transferred to the neurology unit for a few days before finally going to outpatient therapy. She was in a rehab center in Santa Clara, and I visited every Tuesday. She was progressing well, and her speech was improving more rapidly than anyone could have hoped.

But those of you who know my mom know that nothing is easy with her. This was no different. About a month into outpatient therapy she had another stroke.

All of the speech she had regained was obliterated.

Back to the ICU.

When my friends saw that I looked a little puffy-eyed at school, they asked what was wrong. My answer? My mom had to go back to the hospital.

Should I have confided in them and told them how scared I was? Probably. Told them that my mom's entire speech center was now gone? Probably. Told them that they were performing a surgery, essentially in her brain? Probably. Was I too afraid of people thinking I was weak? Definitely.

After the first stroke, I had been getting better at asking for help and letting people in, but nowhere near close enough. On the day of her surgery, I sort of had a breakthrough.

The procedure was supposed to take four hours, and my dad was going to call me when it was done. About five hours after the surgery was scheduled to start, my friends noticed that I seemed, for lack of a better word, off. I was fidgeting, constantly checking my phone, pacing at times, and generally agitated.

My friends pestered me with questions until I broke. It was the first time since my mom's stroke that I told anyone what was truly going on inside her head . . . and inside mine. It felt amazing.

They didn't judge me or think I was weak; instead, they lifted me up from the bottom of the pit. They told me it was going to be OK, that the procedure was probably going off without a hitch, and that I'd see my mom looking phenomenal after school. You know what? They were right.

Granted, she was a little woozy after the blood transfusion, but other than that, she was as fine as she could've been. After that, I started opening up to some of my closer friends. I was still incredibly closed off, but I started taking baby steps.

The miracle is, I didn't feel weaker. I felt free.

Eventually, at sophomore retreat, I took a leap of faith. I confided in my entire grade. All of my classmates embraced me with open arms.

Literally . . .

I think Malik had me in a hug the second I started talking. Even classmates I didn't know well offered me rides and help whenever I needed them. Again, I knew I wasn't being judged or pitied. These people genuinely cared. What a concept, right?

These last two years have been hard, but I'm not afraid to admit that anymore. I'm not afraid to say that, at times, it was all too much.

I'm not afraid to confide in the entire school that I was scared and did need help. And most importantly, I'm not ashamed to admit that I found help. I found it in my teachers, my friends, and all of my classmates at Priory.

My family likes to say, sure, it sucks that mom had a stroke, but why should we dwell on that? We look for the silver linings.

Family time is a higher priority in our lives than it ever has been.

My mom laughs more now.

I never went through the stage that every teenage girl goes through when every conversation with her mom turns into a shouting match.

And I learned to ask for help. I learned that asking for help isn't a sign of weakness but a sign of strength.

When you are able to ask for help, it means you have faith in your relationship with whoever you are asking, that you are in tune with what you need, and that you are strong enough to know that you can't do everything yourself.

As every athlete knows—no matter how much you can bench press, you always need a spotter.

. . .

By the time Sarah finished, Steve and I had gone through about half the box of tissues someone had handed us. Many of my tears were in pain— hearing fully for the first time the suffering she went through because of my stroke, and how much more difficult it made her time in high school. It was painful to realize that our relationship now was almost completely her providing support to me, and not getting any from me.

But there were also tears of joy. Completely unbeknownst to me, our daughter had found a way to bounce forward. She had found a way to grow from the adversity and taught me in the process. Stroke not only changes the lives of survivors but also of those closest to them. It often requires the entire family to recover, adjust, and accept support themselves. Each person in my family has new roles and relationships, and their own part of the recovery journey. My family has rebuilt our family dynamics in this new context.

. . .

"Stroke is a family illness" was the title of the first slide of a
presentation aimed at family members at a four-week intensive speech
therapy program I attended at the Shirley Ryan AbilityLab in Chicago.
It was a central message delivered by the program's director, Professor
Leora Cherney. Each person in the family is affected, of course. She
meant more than this, though. Leora explained that it's equally important
to understand that the family unit itself—the roles and relationships
that define and hold it together—is also deeply impacted. There are new
adversities, responsibilities, and sometimes burdens. Just like an individual
fighting an illness, the family can show resolve, evolve, and sometimes
bounce back stronger for it.

In her work with stroke survivors, health-care professional Gabriele
Kitzmüller and her colleagues identified four common themes in families'
poststroke experiences:[64]

- The family as a lifebuoy
- Absent presence
- Broken foundations
- Finding a new path forward

The first theme, **family as a lifebuoy**, is most notable early, when a
family rallies to get through a trauma. Every member of my family came to
my rescue during and after my stroke, and none more than my mom, Marcia.

Years after my father's death, my mother began dating a man named
Julian. He was also a widower; like my mom he had been deeply in love
with his spouse of many decades. It took quite a few hints before he finally
asked my mom to the movies. We all loved Julian. He treated my mom
well, took Sarah on fishing trips, and was becoming part of the family.

Suddenly, Julian was diagnosed with pancreatic cancer and told he only had a few months to live. About two months later, on a break from her regular turn at his bedside in the hospital, my mom was at home when Steve called to tell her about my stroke and that I was being airlifted from Reno to the Stanford Hospital ICU. Julian didn't have long either. With his supportive kids nearby to continue helping him, my mom took the first flight from Los Angeles to San Francisco. She was waiting for Danny and Sarah when they arrived, repeating to herself, "Come on Steve, get my baby here," when we were in the air bound for Stanford. Within the week, Julian passed away. She flew back to LA for the funeral and then immediately back to be by my side, still in the ICU.

Eight years later, I get choked up when I try to imagine what she went through that week. "It was a very nightmarish time for me, but my focus was Deb," my mom said later. "I never really grieved for Julian until much, much later." In the weeks that followed, when one of us tried to speak words, or in my case make motions, of sympathy and comfort for her, she shrugged it off. Her focus was on helping me and my family. Mom moved north for six months, living in our home to support us full time. She was at times my primary caregiver, often an extra therapist, and a partner to Steve so he could return to work more quickly, and more easily create time for himself. That was so helpful to him and his sanity, and to me because of that.

The second theme, **absent presence**, is what my daughter felt and, thankfully, moved through when her mother disappeared from that role during two of her most formative teenage years. It is the sudden gap created when a family member vacates a role as mother, spouse, or son. Andrea Helft, whose stroke left her exhausted and sleeping much of the time during her early recovery, was confronted with that dynamic when she recovered her energy a bit. Her four-year-old son asked her, "So is this how you're going to be from now on?" She asked, "Do you mean am I going to get older?" He said, "No, are you this way now. Not the mommy who just sleeps all the time." No mom (or dad) wants their kid to perceive them as absent or even requiring support, but often that is the unfortunate reality for younger stroke survivors.

The third theme, **broken foundations**, refers to the collapse of the established family roles which can be overturned in the wake of stroke. The balanced relationships, routines and traditions, mutual support, and specific responsibilities can all be shaken. The emotional duress of stroke can make it incredibly hard to find a way forward. "A lot of marriages just go out the window," shares Dr. Venkat. "It causes a huge amount of strain on a marriage and on a caregiver. When they've studied caregiver stress a year or so after stroke, they find there's a huge level of depression with the caregivers, as well." Like other adversities, Kitzmüller et al. explain, the broken foundations can be rebuilt with the right approach.

Finally, **finding a new path forward** requires effort from all parties and an understanding that roles will be different as the foundations will have changed. The family will have a new identity and dynamic. Psychologist Melanie Drane said, "When one person has survived stroke, in particular with aphasia, the relationships all change, and the voices change, and everything within a family system is renegotiated."

Understanding this is critical. In healthy situations, each person can find a new and healthy role in the family system. After the initial trauma, when all are focused on the survivor and his or her recovery, the family can begin a process of finding a new balance. Family members may feel resentment and treat the changed circumstances as a burden, or they may see this as an opportunity for their own growth as Sarah did. Survivors may dwell on guilt because of roles they are forced to abandon and demand that their loved ones compensate for the deficits, or they can choose to show appreciation and support to those who are stepping up, and work to forge new roles and even stronger relationships.

· · ·

Malik Thoma laments that important relationships have been badly, perhaps irreparably, damaged through his stroke process. He believes that his family bears some blame for the dire outcome of his strokes. He thinks that family members kept information from him during his time in the hospital. While they were trying to look out for him, "I never asked them to do that," he said. At one point, he ordered his mother out of the emergency room. The memory of that brings his mother close to tears. His sister, who is a doctor herself, stepped in to manage his care. She was opposed to having Malik's physicians perform a splenectomy that they believed was necessary. "I became very angry when I found out about this because she really wasn't letting the hematologist do her job. Once I found out what was happening, I said [to my doctors], 'I don't want you to talk to them anymore. I want you to talk to me. I'm the patient.'"

His sister also recommended changes to his medication dosage, which Malik believes may have triggered another stroke. "My relationship with my sister has never been the same because I really feel she overstepped her bounds." Existing problems in the family were only exacerbated. "There's a lot of enmity between my family and my wife," he said. "They can't stand each other, so it's been tough." For Malik, the earliest moments when his family came to support him, to be his lifebuoy, were not handled well, and they have struggled to move past that.

This kind of situation can cause a ripple effect in a survivor's recovery. Effective family involvement and emotional support helps recovery and reduces stress among stroke survivors. Especially as health-care support wanes, it's critical to have a healthy group of people providing care and positivity. Malik has struggled to think positively about many aspects of his recovery, perhaps stemming in part from bitter relationships with those immediately surrounding him.

Mary Jones's husband spent three years as primary caregiver to Mary, providing her support and stability. But he felt unable to find a new path forward that was sustainable for him, so he sent Mary to her family (who put her in a retirement home). The strain many families face is extreme, and it's hard to blame them for being overwhelmed. Julia Fox Garrison put it well. "The patient is the nucleus, and then it ripples out and affects everybody who loves that person 24/7," she said. "Friends and loved ones are all dealing with their own diagnosis; it's called helplessness." In many cases, it requires a full-family effort to work through the crisis.

It is easiest for large families or close communities, which Mary and Malik did not have. Dr. Venkat talked about the Indian community (she is Indian). "Once you have a stroke, they don't leave our stroke patients in facilities. They will always take them home. Sons and daughters and everybody will take turns helping out. The aunts, the uncles, the neighbors, and everyone available will come in and help out. It's a very social thing for us." On the flip side, Dr. Venkat has found that some cultures tend to treat stroke as more shameful, and they isolate those involved, intentionally or implicitly. "In the Korean culture, a very male dominated society, once the man has a stroke and he's become dependent on someone else, that can be the end for him, so to speak." When dependence falls on one person, collapse is far more likely. Support needs to be spread widely among family members.

• • •

In the immediate aftermath of my stroke, Steve inherited roles of primary caregiver, emotional coach, motivator, health-care navigator, financial manager, chief logistician, rehab equipment engineer, and communicator to family, friends, and even my colleagues. It's hard to overstate the demands placed on the partner of a severe stroke survivor. In my situation, I had tremendous resources that other people may not have, and perhaps the greatest is a husband who was willing and able not only to accept the dramatic changes to his life caused by my stroke but also to embrace them fully as part of his life. "Someday we'll look back and this will have been a one-year blip," he'd say often after my stroke. It was always "we," and it was always positive. While I struggled to accept my new deficits and identity, he was already changing his and infusing patience and optimism into our evolving situation.

Each ring supports the next: Steve got support from our kids, my mom, and his family. My in-laws, Marjorie and George Zuckerman, offered many times to come from Boston to help and would have loved to do so. But they and my sister-in-law Marcia accepted Steve's preference not to have more people on-site and instead provided from a distance the emotional support (and distraction from the constant focus on me) that he needed and asked for. They also provided an outlet on the East Coast for our kids, each of whom lived out east for periods following my stroke. "Spouses were convinced that their actions improved the rehabilitation process but emphasized that they, too, needed emotional and practical support," found Kitzmüller, et al. "Support from members of the extended family was crucial. Practical and emotional support allowed spouses to maintain a work life and to keep up with their caregiving obligations during the acute stage."[65] This layer supporting Steve was further removed from the stroke but was critical to our family recovery.

Danny says he thinks he had the least disruption within the family. He was with Steve and me at the time of the stroke, so he saw the damage unfold—terrifying but not the sudden shock that others got. He was going into his senior year at nearby Stanford. "I was in college, and so I had all the distractions in the world to keep me sane," he told me once. "But I was right nearby, so I could visit as often as I wanted to." He leaned on a few good friends and an on-and-off girlfriend, though he says his efforts to accept support were less mature than his younger sister's.

Still, it was a glass-shattering moment for someone who freely admitted to friends that he'd had a blessed life with no real adversity up until then. He may not have known it at the time, but we saw Danny grow up overnight in some dramatic ways. He was suddenly an adult and full partner to Steve during the worst nights, pacing at the hospital, talking through medical options, supporting the rest of the family, and observing therapy sessions. Our relationship had already been moving from mother-son to peers, as all do, and after my stroke, he gracefully accelerated through that evolution.

Adam, our second son, had just started college at Tufts, three thousand miles away. When Steve first told him what was happening, he did what kids his age do—got on the internet to learn about stroke. That both helped and hurt. He could fill in all the uncertainty between calls with Steve and Danny, but usually it confirmed how bad things really were. Fortunately, we could afford to have him fly home whenever he felt the need, so after the stroke he came immediately, and then came home several times in the months following. The first time he came to the hospital to visit, he was shocked. "It was like the rug had been pulled out from under me," he later said of those early weeks and months. "Someone who had cared for me all my life was suddenly incapacitated without warning."

He suggested taking a leave of absence and restarting school in January. I don't remember this, but apparently my nonverbal communication made it crystal clear that was unacceptable to me. He wrestled with it, torn that he wasn't there to know what was going on in real time and to support me when I needed it. He gave in but flew home often in the early months. For two years he only took summer jobs near home to be close.

Meanwhile, Sarah was still living at home. She witnessed my stroke and recovery activities daily through her last three years of high school. As anybody around our family could tell you, Sarah had not been an easy child up to that point. "Deb was always worried about Sarah," remembered Robin Ely. "And she just stepped up. She really grew past some of her challenges." Sarah struggled more when she was younger, really started to find herself in middle school, and in high school was doing well, making new friends, and becoming independent. She was far more responsible than Adam and Danny were at her age.

Sarah drew on soccer and schoolwork and her natural humor. She embraced a new and more adult role, helping me more than I was helping her. Steve stepped into both parenting roles to a degree, and the two of them forged an even closer relationship. Fitness was an important escape and coping mechanism for both of them, and Steve talks about one of the silver linings for him, "How many dads get to do P-90X (a pretty intense video fitness program) in the garage at 6 a.m. with a high school daughter?" Pleasure, health, mutual support, and father/daughter bonding all at once.

Brave as she was, of course Sarah struggled through it, too. "My bad days were [my mother's] bad days—because that was when I really needed to be there for her, those were the hardest. Those were the days I just wanted to run into my room and not deal with it." Just like I had to learn as a survivor, she had to learn it's OK for family to acknowledge the challenge and slip into negativity at times. That's where a family can be so critical—picking each other up in turn. In the eight years since my stroke, whenever our kids are going through school or job transitions, they've talked to each other to make sure one of them stays in the Bay Area; they know that helps both me and Steve.

· · ·

As my family adjusted to support me, our roles were adjusting as well. We were starting to find a new path forward. This is healthy and necessary but can also be painful. Beyond the inconvenience that supporting a survivor causes, it throws family identities into question. If Steve had stepped into both parenting roles, was I no longer a good mother to Sarah? "This psychological, emotional aspect for the stroke survivor and for the family has largely been ignored, but in the last several years, more and more work has been done," said Dr. Venkat. "We now know that the first step is recognition—recognizing that this is a problem. The second step is learning how to fix it." Survivors must wrestle with their own changing role inside their family, which for many of us is a critical aspect of our lives and identities.

Manny Gigante suffered his stroke when he was twenty-nine. He has a very large Filipino family. He had certain expectations about how to be a good father to his boys, and he found himself lacking. "Initially, I struggled with the whole thing about the father's role. But you know, mentoring or parenting my son doesn't necessarily mean I have to be in that physical role. I can coach him in ways to be a good person and a good human being, not just being a good athlete." Manny really wrestled with what it means to be a good father, something that was a powerful part of his identity, but he saw that his stroke didn't have to take that away from him.

Jim Indelicato talked a lot about how life changed for all in his family. He used to be the fixer, the one who could do and did everything. He misses being valued for that. But his daughter Joy understands. "He's just valuable in different ways now." She has helped him see that, too. Rather than being the one who is doing everything, he is coaching and inspiring others. Whether at home or the rehab institute, Jim said, "If I can do this, you can do this." He believes their extremely close family got even closer, but he also feels guilty. "Since the stroke, I feel like two people had a stroke. Me and her. It's not fair for her to have to—" but Diane cut him off. Sure, their husband-and-wife roles have reversed a little, but she also wants to take care of other household things so he can focus on getting better.

Molly Stuart and Tony Hardy are good friends of ours who live in Lake Tahoe. Molly was the first friend on the scene after my stroke. She came to the hospital in Reno while my abilities were still slipping away and later was one of the first to visit me at Valley Medical Center. Their daughter Whitney was four years ahead of Adam at Tufts, and as a four-month-old, she had attended our wedding and amused our mostly single, childless friends by rolling over for the first time. Four years after her graduation, she got engaged to her college boyfriend Dan, and two months after that she went for a winter run in Boston and was struck by a car. She suffered a severe traumatic brain injury (TBI) along with a shattered leg, and fought for her life in the hospital, successfully. But her TBI left her with severe memory loss and other significant cognitive challenges.

After the accident, everybody who cared so much about Whitney immediately came to her aid. Her parents were nearing retirement, but they put everything on hold in California and flew out to Boston to be with her. Dan left his job to be by Whitney's side and help guide her through recovery. Whitney's brother Matt, Dan's family, countless close friends, and extended family all rallied to help Whitney and her support team however possible.

Molly and Tony talked with Dan and told him they would completely understand if he didn't stay in the relationship. This was a life changer, and they didn't think he should stay out of obligation. But he assured them that he'd fallen in love with Whitney and was still in love with her, completely committed to doing whatever it would take. Like Steve for me, he took primary responsibility for managing her care, navigating the medical and insurance quagmire, researching rehabilitation options, and supporting her in every way he could. After almost six months in hospitals, he began to teach her simple tasks like tying her shoes, doing dishes, and folding laundry, and more complicated ones like navigating her way around Boston.

Whitney progressed, and Dan was able to return to work in about a year. They traveled a bit, including to weddings of their friends. They still talked about getting married themselves, but Dan was clear: "We're not having a wedding until I know Whitney will remember it." Optimism and humor are among Dan's many incredible attributes. Things continued to improve. Whitney was becoming a bit more independent. She'd started working part time in simple jobs. They bought a house together. They started to talk about a date for their wedding and began looking for locations on Whitney's home turf near Lake Tahoe.

We were with Molly and Tony at Lake Tahoe when, with tears in their eyes, they shared with us the painful news that the engagement was off. Dan had wrestled for months, but, despite Whitney's significant improvements, he realized he couldn't start the rest of their lives together on a foundation that didn't allow for a true partnership. He explained to Whitney and her parents that more than the physical support she might need, he felt that he could not move forward without a real emotional partner in the relationship, with support flowing both ways. They had been together for almost eight years, and their families had already merged. It wasn't a divorce, but it felt like one.

Whitney returned home to Truckee where Molly and Tony, now retired, had been making plans to rent out their home, outfit an RV, and tour the United States for a bit—a retirement vision they'd had for some time. Change of plans. They reorganized so they could be Whitney's primary support and began to navigate the complex road of finding new doctors and therapists, learning about California disability benefit programs, finding support services, and helping Whitney continue her recovery and build a life consistent with her ongoing disabilities and needs.

Many people have wondered—often out loud with Molly and Tony— whether it would have been easier if Dan had figured out he needed to leave the relationship right away. Would that have saved them all from a second trauma and life adjustment? Molly and Tony don't see it that way at all. "Dan did what was in his heart, and it was a gift to all of us. He was able to give Whitney a kind of support we never could have given her. We have no doubt she has recovered more because he was at her side for those three years, and we were able to close down our business as planned and actually be retired and fully available when Whitney needed us to step up." Whitney is lucky that her family has been able to adapt.

Steve and I have a goal to ride our tandem bike across the country and use it as a chance to talk about stroke awareness, prevention, and recovery. Whitney is signed up to join us if she can, to share the perspective of experiencing life-changing traumatic brain injury in her twenties. Molly and Tony might get that RV after all, and they could lead the cross-country cyclists' support team. Traumas force our plans, like our relationships, to change. But often both can adjust rather than disappear.

. . .

Shortly after Sarah's Chapel Talk in the fall of her senior year, Steve pushed me to step back into the mothering role. For more than two years, I had focused mainly on my recovery. My speech was still limited, and I wasn't doing much to be Sarah's mom. She was doing fine—thank goodness she was so independent—and Steve's a great dad, but it hurt not to be involved.

Sarah had been invited to her senior prom by a guy she didn't know that well, and they had started dating. Sarah had received sex education from school discussions and otherwise, but Steve suggested it was a mother-daughter rite of passage to have The Talk. Despite my limited speech, he pushed me to take the lead, standing by to fill in if necessary. Sarah knew we were having the talk, and we all stood around the island in our kitchen uncomfortably. After about thirty seconds of awkward silence as I gathered the words with all the concentration I could muster, I said:

> *Boyfriend . . . [long pause] . . .*
> > *Yeeessss? (voice rising, half statement, half question)*
> > *. . . [very long pause, eyebrows raised in exclamation, then*
> *rapid explosion of breath and words] . . .*
> > *PREGNANT NO!!!!*

We all erupted in laughter and later agreed that I had just delivered the most efficient mother-daughter talk in history. I'm told by fully fluent friends that they have borrowed my script for their talks. While I know I did not give Sarah any novel information, it was an important moment in our evolving relationship—it was important to me that I could again participate in her life as a mother, and important to her, I think, that she could again see me as a source for advice and guidance as she had before.

STROKE IS A FAMILY ILLNESS: CHAPTER 9 HIGHLIGHTS

- Stroke will impact the lives of everybody in the immediate family, both initially and long-term.
- The family unit can navigate this change together, not just providing support to the survivor but also renegotiating roles and norms over time.
- Family members will likely face their own challenges and can also grow from this journey.
- Survivors may have to come to terms with changing roles, like redefining what it means to be a good parent or child.

CHAPTER 10.

Partners and Intimacy

About six months after my stroke, some tension started to build in my relationship with Steve. My extreme physical dependency was gone, and my mom had returned to her home in Los Angeles. I could navigate the house, get my own food, and I had just started to take driving lessons in a car equipped with a left foot gas pedal and a knob on the wheel so I could steer one-handed. My days were pretty much organized around doing as much outpatient therapy as insurance would support, with lots of self-therapy, too—very slow walks and efforts to exercise in the gym. Steve was back at work full time. Although he had built more flexibility into his schedule and was certainly supporting me a lot, in some ways he was getting back to his old life. I most certainly was not.

Steve would come home, and I'd have a mental list of all the things I couldn't do during the day and wanted him to help with. Of course, it was hard to communicate what I wanted, and in the frustration of trying, I'd frequently get pissed off at him. When we were together, and he jumped up to get something he could tell I wanted, I'd get mad that he was treating me as if I couldn't do things for myself. I was trying so hard not to be dependent. When I tried to do something for myself, like getting a cup of coffee that ended up all over the floor, I'd get pissed that he hadn't offered to help. Doors were a great cause of friction. If he rushed to open them, I'd glare at him as if saying, "You didn't think I could do that myself?" But if he didn't help, and I struggled, my look would say, "I had a fucking stroke, want to help me out here?"

Of course, I wasn't really mad at Steve; I was mad at my situation. But Steve is my partner, and he was close by, so he became the target. It was irrational, particularly since he was such a rock as my most essential supporter, but emotions are not rational. Steve was incredibly patient, but understandably, he resented my attacks. Sometimes he would withdraw. "At times I would think, 'Screw this—whatever I do is wrong, so I just won't try so hard,'" Steve said later. This dynamic took its toll. Anger, resentment, withdrawal, then more anger, more resentment, more withdrawal—it was inevitable that the partnership would begin to spiral downward if we didn't find a better path forward.

Those were the early signs of our broken foundations. Thankfully, we had a strong foundation and lots of support. We had pulled out of downward spirals before and found new paths in other situations. But it still hasn't been easy. A stroke will challenge the pair not just in caregiving, but in every aspect of the partnership: the balance of emotional support, roles within the family and household, financial responsibility, attitudes, and yes, sex. My personal identity and my partnership with Steve have evolved, as they must for every stroke survivor.

• • •

Immediately after a stroke, nearly all focus is on the survivor. But the demands on those closest to them, often their spouse or partner, are incredibly strenuous. "Role changes and altered relationships made the healthy spouses face responsibilities with which they were unfamiliar. These role changes often caused fear and insecurity or interfered with work obligations,"[66] wrote Kitzmüller and her colleagues. Often, supporters don't have nearly as much help as they need. Not only are they the primary caregiver, they are also constantly on call, deprioritizing their own desires, trying to emotionally support the survivor, and putting the other parts of their life on hold.

Faced with physical challenges, caregiving needs, and emotional stress, Julia Fox Garrison talked of how hard it was to appreciate the strains on her husband and find a good path forward. Particularly in the first year, there were trying times that tested their marriage. One of the biggest challenges was the terrible mood swings caused by some of the medication Julia was taking. "One minute I'd be saying, 'I love you, I love you,' and the next minute I'd be screaming, 'You're a jerk.' It was just whacked. But he was so strong." Fortunately, Jim saw through that kind of anger. Julia calls Jim her rock, and he jokingly calls Julia his hard place.

Relationships are complicated. They are difficult. They require a lot of work to make them strong even without the stress of a stroke or another traumatic, life-changing event. In the United States, almost 50 percent of all marriages end in divorce or permanent separation.[67] After a stroke, it is only natural to expect that relationships will require even more work to evolve and thrive.

Of course, those survivors who face their recovery without a partner have an even harder road. I cannot imagine having gone through this journey without Steve. Those of us with partners often count on them to be our biggest allies—further reason to appreciate how this partnership can evolve after stroke.

. . .

Malik Thoma has had a difficult time navigating his relationship post stroke. When I asked how the stroke had affected his relationship with his wife, he replied, "Devastating." She lives with her parents now, and Malik lives with his mother, who is most involved in his recovery. "My wife and I have a very different relationship," he explained. "She's very angry at me still, four years later."

As Malik talked about his marriage, it became clear that significant problems had existed in their relationship before his stroke. She was angry at him for taking the risk of starting a business rather than staying in a stable job. She is a very religious woman, and she was angry that his entrepreneurial efforts required that he work on Saturdays, the Muslim Sabbath. She was also angry that he was living under so much stress at work, thinking it made him a less attentive husband and father. The stroke and the stress of life in recovery seemed to amplify their preexisting marital challenges, rather than serving as an opportunity to deliberately reexamine the relationship.

Malik's wife's reactions are understandable. A loved one's stroke can alter the course of a spouse's life almost as much as the person affected, and it is common to feel some resentment. Although neither Malik nor his wife ever said they were separated, their descriptions of the life they shared made it sound as if they were. They seem to be stuck resenting each other, rather than working to find a new path forward in the changed reality.

A study of survivors and their families by Kitzmüller and colleagues revealed that it is relatively common for relationships to fold under the stress of poststroke life. Previous relationship troubles or a shorter relationship— less than five years—made it far likelier that the relationship would dissolve after stroke. "In most of these cases either the survivor didn't want to limit the partner's life, or the healthy partner was unwilling to build a future together that would incorporate the survivor's disabilities and resultant changes to their previously anticipated roles in the relationships."[68] Mary Jones's husband supported her for three years, but they never truly found a sustainable partnership or path forward. After three years, he filed for divorce and sent her home to family in St. Louis.

Sometimes it goes the other way. Two of the men in the study by Kitzmüller and her colleagues moved out to live on their own in order to save their wives from the obligations of survivor support. They didn't end their relationships; they visited regularly and spent holidays together. Their moves were not purely altruistic; the study's authors wrote, "Independence was of such importance that they decided to live on their own."

• • •

Julia Fox Garrison wrestled with changing roles from the very beginning. In sharing her story, she told me, "My husband had become a nurse to take care of me. I couldn't even be a wife, and so I went through this identity crisis about who I was." She did a lot more thinking after that early crisis, realizing there were a lot of different ways to be a wife.

Julia really helped me see how the survivor's recognition and deliberate effort can be critical to supporting partners. In the second year after her stroke, she recognized that their relationship was increasingly defined by her being the patient and Jim the caregiver, and she knew things needed to change. "I made a conscious decision on this one particular day," Julia told me. She said to Jim, "That's it. The stroke is taking a backseat. It's not going to be at the steering wheel anymore. I want you to be married to me because you're happy and having fun and we're a partnership. I don't want you to be married to me because you're stuck, because you have to be my nurse. I don't want you to be my nurse. I want you to be my husband." With a broad smile, she finished, "That's when things started getting better with our relationship."

Kitzmüller and her colleagues described the situation for other couples much like Fox Garrison: "Together, they had to rearrange their lives and adjust to the changes that had broken their foundation." Stroke recovery does not need to define the relationship, but it can contribute to its strength. Time spent together on therapy can be a source of bonding, and there is value in participating in peer groups that expand support networks to people with common stroke experiences. "After some time, the changes in marital life became routine," the researchers observed. "Couples did not reflect much on the past; rather, they wanted to look forward . . . Their strategy was to focus on opportunities rather than on limitations."[69]

Rose Miller, wife of aphasic stroke survivor Randy Miller, shared the same forward-thinking attitude when it came to her husband's stroke recovery.

But the couple had to make a concerted effort to move beyond the caregiver–patient dynamic to ensure a healthy basis for their marriage. In an effort to restore some balance to the relationship, Rose chose to use the term "care partner" instead of "caregiver." To her, it is not a matter of one giving and the other receiving. She believes they are in the battle of stroke recovery together. "It's not one of us; it's both of us," she said.

Deidre Warren was in the final years of a long career as a registered nurse at a cardiac rehabilitation hospital when a stroke literally knocked her down in the street outside her church. Mike, her husband of forty-four years, had retired just six months before her stroke, and the couple has two grown sons, both serving in the U.S. Air Force. When her younger son Deron flew home from Germany with his family upon hearing about her stroke, he packed his dress blues because he didn't know if he might be going to his mother's funeral.

Despite her incredible work ethic, Deidre's physical disabilities remain significant. While she has no aphasia, she's not very independently mobile. She can walk with a cane and brace, but a wheelchair is far more practical. Two years after her stroke, her husband Mike still goes wherever she goes. He gets up most nights to help Deidre go to the bathroom, and he does the hard work of loading her wheelchair into the car, cooking, shopping, cleaning, and providing care in every shape and form. Their family vacations and shared retirement look very different now from what they had envisioned.

Mike talked very openly about how much life has changed and how he has dealt with it. "All the time, different types of anger," he said. "The anger resulting from frustration, taking that out on her. When I reflect back, it's probably 80 percent on my shoulders. It wasn't her fault. It was the stroke's fault." His anger is not at Deidre but the situation. In fact, some of it is on her behalf—disappointment about the loss of time spent with her kids.

Mike is with his wife nearly every minute of every day, joined at the hip by her dependence. But he feels grateful that he has the ability to help her. As they explored a new marital path together with Mike as Deirdre's care partner, Mike found himself rediscovering what made him fall in love with his wife in the first place. "The same thing that is frustrating—being together for twenty-four hours a day, seven days a week—is also one of the nice things," he said. "You're remembering why you fell in love all over again," Deidre teased.

. . .

Early on, Steve got good advice; he'd be no good as support for me if he didn't take care of himself. That also meant I had to do what I could to take care of him and the rest of the family over this long journey. I looked for small gestures of appreciation, even if they weren't always eloquent. These matter to the people around you. In a study of nurse practitioners in analogous caregiving situations, a team of researchers found that, "At the front line, NPs worked day by day to secure small wins, such as special 'thank yous' from patients and even minor recognition of their knowledge and skills . . . small wins generated confidence that energized continued work toward new roles."[70]

Rose Miller told me that despite Randy's severe aphasia, he ordered flowers for her online and had them delivered to the house to celebrate their anniversary without her knowing. "That was a light bulb moment," she said. "There've been those kind of moments throughout the whole time, and you think, 'Oh. OK. The love, caring, and appreciation are still there.'" Randy's personality clearly remains and is increasingly revealed as he continues improving.

Steve and I spoke with his former classmate, Art Varnado, and his wife Martina, after a recent class reunion. Martina has struggled with a loss of balance in her relationship with Art as the impact of her multiple sclerosis becomes more severe. Martina and Art had worked hard to have a real partnership in marriage. They both worked full time in professional roles, and with two daughters at home (until one left for college recently) they shared parenting and other home responsibilities. Martina talked about how much she appreciates all that Art and Marla, their daughter still in high school, do to help her. So it really bothers her when they have to do her half of the household work. It challenges her identity as a partner. So she will occasionally ask her sister or a friend or hire someone to take care of what she used to do so that it doesn't fall on Art. It's not economically feasible for everyone, but it's another form of recognizing the changing roles in a partnership and finding creative ways to address them.

I have found that sometimes the most helpful support I can provide to Steve is giving him the space and encouragement to do the things that make him happy, without me. Every time he goes off on a long bike ride, or skiing with friends, or to a party that I know will be loud and too frustrating for me to enjoy, it hurts because I used to love those things, too. But I know we'll all be better off in the long run if I don't ask him to give up all those things just because I can't participate with him in the same way anymore.

We haven't seen a counselor or sought other professional help since my stroke, but we do draw on relationship-management tools from having had counseling twice before. Ten years into our marriage, we were juggling life with three young kids, and both of us faced the pressure of intense, demanding careers that were very important to us. Stress and tension were building, and we were lucky to cross paths with Learning as Leadership (LAL), a personal and professional training and development group that helped us learn to better manage stress in our relationship. A bit later, about five or six years before my stroke, we hit another rough patch and had several visits with a counselor recommended by a friend. Those sessions were incredibly helpful then, and they left us with insights and tools that have helped us stay connected during the poststroke period.

• • •

One important part of our strong relationship is sex, as it is for many couples. Although sex certainly isn't the only form of intimacy that makes our relationship rewarding, it is an important one. Based on several dozen conversations and a bit of research, I think I am something of a lucky exception. For me, sex improved after my stroke, pretty much immediately. I really don't know why. It's a silver lining I allow myself to enjoy.

An article called "Sex and Intimacy after Stroke," by Jon Caswell, published on the website of the American Stroke Association includes the following: "Where the stroke happens in the brain determines how the survivor is affected. If a stroke occurs in the frontal lobe, the survivor may be less aware of socially appropriate behavior and feel less inhibited."[71] That's not where my stroke happened, so it's not my source of good fortune. Steve has guessed that, "All the stress was forced out of you." Before my stroke, I was always a bit wound up and stressed; now I live more in the moment, so I can get out of my own head and really enjoy the experience. Of course, some of the practicalities have changed. I'm less agile than I used to be. We have to be careful of my right arm and hand, still with limited capabilities. But only the most extreme disabilities, which fortunately I don't have, are a physical obstacle to a healthy sexual relationship. The real barriers are generally emotional and psychological, and fortunately, those haven't been an issue for me.

Unfortunately, I seem to be in the minority on this. A UK study reported that among stroke survivors under fifty years of age, sexual difficulty rates were much higher than those found in the general population, which runs at 40 percent for women and 30 percent for men.[72] Caswell frames the challenge well: "Stroke-related physiological and psychological changes may affect both sexual desire and performance. The insecurity, fear, and doubt that can arise from this can throw even the most open and loving couples into a tangled web of conflicting emotions for both sides: Is sex safe? Am I still attractive? Can I be both a caregiver and a lover?"[73] Experts and survivors alike agree that in most cases, there is no reason all of these issues cannot be overcome so that couples can re-create a very healthy sex life.

Several stroke survivors I talked to struggled with body image issues. Andrea Helft, an avid recreational athlete in her early forties at the time of her stroke, is another survivor for whom body image was a real barrier. Changes to her capabilities and appearance impacted her self-image, and spending time in therapy groups with people who were often twice her age further stripped away any feelings of being young and vivacious. She knew that physically, she could return to intimacy, but her opinion of herself got in the way. She just felt old and unattractive and, therefore, not inclined. Andrea explained with regret, "I have no interest at all in sex. None. For a long time, it was because I was simply too tired. I just was asleep. I couldn't stay awake. Then . . . I don't even know. I think it's all wrapped up in this not feeling young and vital and the whole thing. I just have no desire."

Julia also had to overcome problems before restarting her sex life. "How could I feel very attractive?" she asked. "I'm not even connected to my body." She had to stay open-minded to new possibilities, accept herself as she was, and never give up on herself. Even then, there were physical challenges. Initially, sex felt like a weight-lifting session for both Julia and Jim. But it was important to both of them to reconnect sexually as a couple, so they kept trying. Julia figured out that since her brain didn't know she had a left side, she had to use her eyes to compensate. About a year after her stroke, they tried leaving all the lights on so she could see where her left hand and arm were during sex. Over time it got better, as they tried new things and learned strategies that made it more enjoyable. "We don't have the overhead lights on anymore," Julia told me. "Now we use candles, which helps us get in the mood."

Rose Miller, talking for both herself and for her survivor husband Randy because of his severe aphasia, was clear about the continued strength of their relationship. She talked about a close bond they feel in every activity they do together, whether its mowing the lawn or making love. Of sex, she said,

"Obviously you have to change things with the physical limitations, but we don't seem to have a problem with that." Sitting next to Randy, she turns to him with a little smile. "What do you think?" Randy nods emphatically and smiles back at her. "Yeah," he said simply. Aphasia has robbed him of words, but the meaning was clear.

The fondness between Randy and Rose, both in their midfifties when I met them, is obvious. That close bond she described was so clear as we just sat and talked. Sex is part of their relationship, but another kind of intimacy is also apparent, which is consistent with the findings of Meghann Jane Grawburg, a researcher in the field of speech and language sciences at the University of Canterbury in New Zealand. Grawburg interviewed more than one hundred stroke survivors with aphasia and their spouses. They reported less frequent sexual intimacy, but she found that it was often replaced by other forms of physical intimacy. With one partner having limited speech capacity, affection was often shown with increased physical touching during normal activities, instead of verbal expressions of love.[74]

Gail Rusch's story illustrates how important our partner's role is in this area. After her stroke, Gail did not feel at all attractive, was not interested in sex, and was afraid her partner was upset that sex was no longer part of their relationship. She had been with her sweetheart, as she endearingly called him, for fifteen years, although they were not married. She didn't want him to feel trapped and unhappy, so she told him that he didn't have to stay with her, and he could go be with a woman who could give him everything he wanted. He told her that he loved her, as she was and as she is. He was happy right where he was. "I had very low confidence when it came to my womanhood," Gail said. "But he changed my mind when he told me that." This is such a clear reminder that so many things in our lives, even sex, are driven not by our capabilities but by our sense of self, our identity, and that our identity is powerfully influenced by those around us, especially those closest to us.

• • •

Aphasia presents the biggest ongoing challenge in my partnership with Steve. When I want to communicate, I frequently have trouble getting my message out; just listening to me requires more patience. My increased brevity makes me sound more impatient than I really feel. Or a particularly emotive response may come across as angry. And on Steve's side, the added stress and responsibility of poststroke life can lead him to snap in frustration a bit more than he used to.

Kitzmüller and her colleagues wrote about a dynamic that resonated with us:

> *Stroke survivors with severe aphasia had to rely on their spouses as interpreters, although their interpretations were not always correct. It was obvious during the interviews with couples that aphasic stroke survivors wanted to talk on their own behalf but had difficulties entering the conversation. Sighs and groans were uttered when the spouse dominated the conversation. Spouses of stroke survivors who had completely lost their speech abilities were forced to make guesses that caused misunderstandings and conflicts.[75]*

Some of what has helped Steve and my relationship stay strong through all the stress is simply good luck. Steve is by nature a "look forward, not back" person. According to his mom, "It is what it is," was one of his favorite expressions as a kid. He has treated my stroke as a bump in the road, one of life's twists we simply must deal with. That is not my nature, as I often feel determined to control my own fate. His ability to deal with our new reality with a positive attitude and problem-solving approach has been a huge blessing for me. And he said that if I were more passive about life after stroke, he would have a much harder time being as supportive as he is. Whether it was luck or attraction that drew us together, that compatibility helps in everything we do together, including sex.

Even so, we continue to have plenty of challenges working on our partnership. Ironically, one of the things that sometimes drives me crazy is Steve's overwhelmingly positive attitude—the same positive attitude I usually appreciate so much. Sometimes when I'm struggling and giving myself permission to be angry at the world, his eternal positivity makes it seem as if he's oblivious to the very real struggles I, we, still have. My reaction depends on my mood, the narrative I'm in, and what else is going on around me. Likewise, the way Steve responds to my inconsistent reactions depends on his stress level at the time. Thankfully, we work through issues honestly and together, continuing to forge a new path forward in a different and always-evolving partnership.

PARTNERS AND INTIMACY: CHAPTER 10 HIGHLIGHTS

- This chapter focuses on survivors who have a spouse or partner; not all do, and recovery can be even more difficult without the critical support a partner can provide.
- The balance of partnerships is nearly always changed after stroke.
- This can be extremely onerous for the supporting partner and can make the survivor feel like a burden; it is important to talk about these realities and renegotiate expectations.
- Some marriages and partnerships do fail, but many emerge even stronger and more rewarding than before.
- Sex lives can be just as fulfilling after stroke as before, though sex often requires acknowledging and overcoming some physical or mental barriers.

CHAPTER 11.

People Are Social Animals

Seven months after my stroke, one of my good friends, Anne Payne, was organizing a girls' trip to celebrate her fiftieth birthday. The plan was for a weekend of fun in the sun in Palm Springs, California. This is an active group of women: runners, hikers, bikers, swimmers, and avid tennis players. Conversations are lively and the fun gets loud. At first, I said I couldn't go, as I had for so many other things since my stroke. I could barely walk without holding someone's arm, and my speech was still almost nonexistent. Joining them would clearly be an exercise in frustration and jealousy.

One of my closest friends and part of the group, Kim Menninger, argued with me. She offered to help with anything I needed, from the logistics of travel to putting in my contacts. She said she'd help make space for me to have fun, whatever that meant, and whatever that took. Nervously, I decided to give it a shot.

I wanted so much to be the "old Deb" that weekend. At the airport, I was determined to get through TSA security on my own with no help. Kim told me later that when I got through to the gate successfully, I was beaming in a way she hadn't seen before. I did know there would be lots of compromises and lots of help needed, but it was good to prove to myself that I could do something on my own.

Once there, frustration was constant. Conversation moved too quickly for me to catch up and contribute. Friends suggested words more quickly than I'd like when I had trouble finding them. I couldn't participate in many activities and at times felt I was holding the group back. Yet, it felt fantastic to be with the group, soaking up the energy of friendship. Kim helped, or just hung back, whenever needed. I went for some nice slow walks, spent a little time in the pool. And at the actual birthday party, I got up and danced for the first time since my stroke.

It wasn't even close to the old me, but spending fun time with women who'd made my life special before the stroke reminded me how powerful good friends and a sense of belonging are to my well-being. It made me realize how much I'd been limiting myself by hesitating to rejoin the social world.

. . .

Our close relationships and interactions with those around us play a huge role in shaping who we are and, even for the introverts among us, guiding our satisfaction. The second level in Maslow's pyramid includes the need for a sense of belonging. As David Brooks wrote, we are *The Social Animal*.[76] Lab experiments, prison studies, and war stories all tell us that people who are completely isolated quickly begin to lose their sanity. "We appear to stand alone, but we are manifestations of relatedness," psychologist Kenneth Gergen said.[77] Our identities are not created by ourselves alone. They are socially constructed. We learn what we value and validate who we are by the relationships and communities we are a part of.

Yet despite its importance to our mental well-being, virtually all stroke survivors I know with substantial disabilities are at least somewhat reluctant to rejoin some of the social structures they enjoyed before their strokes or to build new ones. In a study of young stroke survivors, Dr. Kerry Kuluski and colleagues found that many participants distanced themselves from social relationships and outings. Some did so because it was a reminder of their former selves. Others were worried that they would be perceived as withdrawn and not fun anymore or too self-absorbed. Others impacted by memory loss or inability to engage in meaningful conversation just didn't see the point.[78] Many of the activities we had participated in before might be difficult or impossible now. Being close to them might cause painful longing for what once was.

There are many fair reasons to feel anxiety. Our disabilities can make social interaction difficult, and the emotional trauma and confusion can make us unsure about previous relationships. Additionally, survivors may feel they are burdening friends by forcing them to cope with their disability. So, for some survivors, friendships can actually feel like a negative factor rather than a source of strength. In one study, Dr. Jennifer Guise argues, ". . . sufferers may be more concerned about their changed roles and relationships than recovery of physical function."[79] For some, this may cause a temporary or partial hesitation, but for others it can lead to a full retreat from pre-stroke social circles.

It is true that we are forced to reckon with the fact that in some ways, we may be an additional burden on those around us. Family and friends may be forced to alter some activities, repeat certain things, wait patiently while we fight through our impaired speech, or even provide emotional support as we struggle through such a taxing time. But in my own experience and with those interviewed for this book, I have found that close friends are usually not only willing to help and be patient, they also relish the opportunity to do so. Having a friend like Kim, eager to provide help whenever I needed it as she did for the girls' trip, helped me push through my hesitancy to rejoin my social circle, which has been instrumental in my recovery.

• • •

Andrea Helft was in her early forties at the time of her stroke. She still struggles with significant memory issues and pain, but thankfully, her energy has returned. She has embraced Dr. Kuluski and colleagues' "quest narrative" in her recovery, charting out a path to find a poststroke identity. Her network rallied behind her immediately, supporting both her and her family. "The incredible emotional support from our friends and family. They were really awesome," said her husband Ryan of the beginning of their journey. After the initial wave of support, Andrea and her friends were left to confront very new circumstances and the reality of her stroke.

"My stroke rattled some of my friends," she said. Andrea had always defined herself largely by her work and by being a high achiever. Now that was taken away, and she was struggling just to stay awake. She had aphasia and it was difficult to remember questions that were asked of her just seconds before. Her friends thought about their own values and priorities, spurred on by Andrea's trauma.

A few of her closest friends joined her in wellness classes designed to help them think through what truly brings them joy in life. "We've been doing a lot of work together around meditation and mindfulness," said Andrea. Rather than facing these big, scary questions alone, Andrea and her friends have been tackling them together. The experience has made them all closer as friends. Andrea has realized that friends and relationships are actually her priority and are at the core of her identity now, much more important than being a high achiever. "For me, that's a big shift," she said.

This journey has made Andrea not only thankful for her friends but in some ways for her stroke. She's found incredibly rich silver linings because the stroke has helped her shift her values to be more focused on family and close friends. "It's like a ball of warmth that I have," she said. "Not only deeper connections with my friends but an understanding that they're really there for me when things are bad." Her friends were more than a support network when things got bad, and she realized they were an important part of her life and identity.

As a product of helping Andrea with her recovery, two of her best friends have gained some clarity themselves. They have achieved what Sandberg and Grant referred to as "pre-traumatic growth"—learning from being adjacent to a trauma, rather than actually going through one directly.

It is cliché for a trauma or major life event to provide a "wake-up call" to those surrounding the most affected, "putting things in perspective." Unfortunately, this is often a temporary change before we settle back into routines. Letting friends and others be part of the post-trauma journey and challenges can be a blessing rather than a burden, allowing them to learn from the experience and gain long-term perspective as well.

. . .

I knew I had close friends who would support and not judge me, and yet I still hesitated to be social. Especially with aphasia, the barriers to active conversation and social engagement were real. I was self-conscious when I presented my severe disabilities for the first time. I knew I should meet with people and be confident, but I just wasn't. Sean Maloney, a friend and fellow survivor who also has speech challenges, sent me an email reflecting just that struggle:

> *I was an extrovert, now I am an introvert.*
> *I used to stun an audience with my wit, now I am in the audience,*
>   *watching, skeptical.*
> *I used to be so famous, now I am jaded. I have seen it all before.*
> *Get a life!*
> *I should be more of an extrovert!*
>
> *– Sean*

Nearly every stroke survivor I talked to had initial difficulties in rebuilding a social life. The challenges faced vary depending on the person and the disability, so the strategy for how best to reintegrate with friends will vary as well. There are six reasons for social hesitation that I've encountered most frequently. In each case, survivors have found ways to embrace the challenges and have emerged with friendships that are as strong as ever.

1. I PHYSICALLY CAN'T BE SOCIAL

You can!

Yes, our physical and speech constraints make it harder. Some of our former activities may be impossible now, and some relationships based on those bonds may not recover. But if we are willing to adapt and look forward, any of us can have a meaningful group of friends and social life.

Of all the survivors I've gotten to know, Laure Wang clearly has the most physical constraints. She is confined to a wheelchair and unable to move anything but her eyes. Her social life has changed dramatically. But after several years, she realized she could do far more than she first thought she could. After initially saying she wouldn't be there, she decided to go to a school reunion. Her friend Fabiola said, "I felt like that weekend changed Laure's attitude toward adjusting to her new life." Everyone was thrilled to see her, and she was outgoing, laughing, and enjoying her old friends—even if it was in a very new way. "It showed she's still the same outgoing person she always was."

2. IT'S TOO HARD TO BE WORTH IT

Like so many things after a stroke, socializing is harder. This can be incredibly frustrating, and it may mean fewer interactions with new people. But it absolutely does not need to rob us of critical social interactions in our quest to rebuild an identity in the face of our changed life.

Gail Rusch is an African-American woman who was a customer-service trainer by profession and also coached people wanting to run their first marathon. Fifty-three years old and the picture of health when her stroke occurred, she lost both her ability to work and to run and coach running. She lost many of the relationships that centered around her previously physical and active lifestyle. She simply couldn't engage the way she used to. In her late fifties, her mobility did improve, but it was still impaired, both physically and with speech difficulties due to her aphasia. A huge piece of her identity and social life was gone.

"I finally decided to rebuild myself from the inside out," Gail said. She enrolled in Alameda Junior College, and then transferred to California State University to study human development and family studies. She graduated in June 2016. "I had to think really hard about how I felt. Then I would slowly start to bring myself out, you know? It was a slow but steady process." Gail feels that going to school, a huge and challenging step, was a catalyst in the process of recreating her identity. That hard work has paid off. Her social life now, albeit more challenging than before, seems normal to her again. Now, "I can't remember how I was treated when I didn't have [a stroke]," she said.

Once we commit ourselves to looking forward and creating a meaningful social life, we realize how many ways we can adapt. My speech is better in the morning than in the evening when I'm tired, so we try to invite people over for brunch, not dinner. Loud restaurants are difficult, so we often bring burritos home from the neighborhood cantina and enjoy food and friendship in the quiet of our home. When I turned sixty, I told Steve I didn't want a party, but I did have four birthday celebrations with small groups of family or friends. I now practice meditation, sneaking off for twenty minutes to calm myself and reenergize if things get overwhelming at an outing. And I'm simply more selective about social engagements to keep enough energy for those I choose to join.

3. OTHER PEOPLE PISS ME OFF

Laure Wang initially avoided most social interaction. She hated the pity she saw in the eyes of those around her. It is hard to miss Laure when she enters the room. She arrives in a wheelchair with a family member, friend, or caretaker always by her side to help navigate and communicate. Sometimes there was overt hostility, but mostly it was nonverbal clues that she was not welcome. Of course, she didn't know what they were really thinking, but she knew how she felt—and she couldn't stand it.

Over time, Laure learned to care less about curious eyes. She has more acceptance of her locked-in condition and that she can't control how other people feel in her presence. She decided she needed to live for herself again. She wrote, "I became bolder, and my mantra was, 'If you don't ask, you will never get.'" She began to own her condition and be more active asking others to make accommodations where necessary. Enjoying cocktails at a local bar one evening, she spotted baseball legend Alex Rodriguez (A-Rod) and decided to ask for a photo with him. "I realized I didn't need much courage to ask. After all, who can say no to a woman in a wheelchair?"

4. I'M A BOTHER

Along with the frustration at our lack of independence, many of us feel extreme insecurity about the burden we place on those we depend on. After the initial wave of support, the journey of stroke recovery is a long one, and it changes the balance of relationships. Intimate families have decades of bonds, not to mention the evolutionary inclination to care for kin, to hold them together as they navigate these changes. With friends, those bonds are not as strong or unconditional. It's easy to fear that perhaps our presence is more of a burden than a joy. As my close friends Kim Menninger and Lizzie Bradley—and so many more—have shown me, our fears are often groundless, and we hold on to them far longer than we should.

Trish Hambridge has always had a large group of friends. She said she now knows who her close friends truly are and those who are only friends "in the past tense." Some struggled to deal with her aphasia more, and she does see them less now. "I'm a little bit disappointed in the way that group kind of dwindled away to some extent," said her father Doug. That is natural as the journey moves from support to social life, though. Trish now focuses her social attention on her closer friends.

For stroke survivors, social interaction takes more effort. We should be more selective with who we spend time with. Trish always valued having a wide circle of friends, but now that this is harder, she takes steps to reduce the burden on everyone. She'll schedule chats on Skype or pull people together in groups herself. And she'll reach out to others with aphasia who can all communicate with full understanding.

Perhaps most important, she still has an active social life and strong friendships with those who are closest to her. "She's the best friend ever, but it's different," said Trish's friend Delia. "Trish is a friend whom you can tell anything to. She will give you good advice. Now I'm also a good friend to her, and I wasn't before." Friendships change, but many of us find that those closest to us are even more supportive than before.

5. I'M EMBARRASSED

When I asked Malik Thoma about his friends, he looked away. Searching for something positive to say, he explained that he does have one good friend, Ron, whom he meets with every so often. But he tells me that he mostly avoids his old friends and former colleagues. "I'm very ashamed of the fact that I'm really not doing that much," he said. He feels a bit embarrassed when Ron asks him what he's up to.

Malik struggles to look at his life without comparison to what he was before. It warps how he interacts with others because he projects feelings onto them that they may not have. His wife is frustrated by how much he has curtailed his social life since the stroke. "The Amazon guy knows about his stroke," she said. "Every time, he can't help it. It's the first thing he presents about himself."

He has let himself be embarrassed by his new circumstance, when he could choose instead to embrace a new social identity. This is not easy. But just as Laure has chosen to care less about the pity she sees in people's eyes when she enters a room, Malik might have a more positive poststroke life if he found a way to care less about the perceptions of others and any embarrassment this may cause him.

6. I'M DEPRESSED

One in three stroke survivors suffers some degree of depression, even if it's never diagnosed. And every survivor I know, even if not clinically depressed, has had periods of extreme frustration that leave them in a rut, feeling isolated and down. Unfortunately, this can be self-reinforcing, with initial feelings of isolation leading to the desire to withdraw ourselves more. Of course, that can lead to more isolation and a downward spiral.

For any survivors with deep clinical depression, some of the strategies that have helped me and other survivors may simply not work. Depression is a serious illness and deserves focused medical assistance. But for many of us, some deliberate strategies can really help.

One of the most important ways to push through mild depression is an active social life. Studies consistently show that social networks lead to increased well-being and health. Knowing this and making an effort to find comfortable ways to engage with friends can be enough to break the downward spiral. Randy Miller has had bouts with depression, and he said, "It's a roller coaster. It's up and down." It's often very hard to take the first steps to break the cycle, whether aided by antidepressants or not.

Randy and his wife Rose started their own aphasia Meetup group that gets together to talk every week. Through the group, they've made some new friends. They go out for dinner and lunch together twice a week, and sometimes they play cards. Randy loves the group and enjoys practicing speech in this safe zone. It has allowed both Randy and Rose to continue engaging socially, even though their social identity has shifted.

One strategy I've used was inspired by my daughter Sarah. She's generally an upbeat, positive kid, but, like most of us, she occasionally needs to vent. One day when Steve was encouraging her not to complain and suggesting ways to solve the problem, she asked, "Can't we just have a five-minute pity party?" Sure, why not? When I'm feeling particularly down, I try to recognize that need to give myself a little time to feel down and angry about my stroke, ideally with Steve or someone else very close to me who knows that it's a short-term strategy, not the beginning of a longer-term slide. When time is up, I can appreciate having given myself space to acknowledge the bad stuff, and it usually helps me refocus on looking forward.

. . .

"Identities are not simply features or products of the individual," wrote Dr. Guise and her colleagues. They "should be viewed as practices with others and the outcomes of those interactions."[80] After stroke, we are in a process of rebuilding our sense of self and navigating a changing identity. Despite new barriers, it's crucial for us to find ways to be social. We can only understand our changing identities through these experiments and interactions. In "Social Identity and Stroke," Sharon Anderson and Kyle Whitfield wrote, "Social relationships are the foundation upon which survivors rebuild skills to engage with the world."[81]

Of course, friends are critical for providing support to a survivor after stroke. But their role extends far beyond that. As survivors recover from a stroke, they are reevaluating their social identity: who they are in the context of others. Some friends will adjust to the new circumstances, while others will give stroke survivors a sense of stability by maintaining their pre-stroke attitudes. In one study, a participant "made a direct link between how friends positioned her as the person she had always been, rather than as disabled and different from that earlier self." This participant said, "They don't look at me like there's something different," which stood out compared with others she was not as close to. She stressed the fact that her most supportive friends reaffirmed her usual identity, rather than her impairments and differences."[82] Both are important: seeing the differences in how friends act helps us determine what relationships and interactions we want and need going forward.

Identity scholar Laksmhi Ramarajan said this type of friendship is critical to and welcomed by many stroke survivors. When rebuilding a new identity, she recommended, "Find a small community where you can test out and experiment with a new behavior. You need some way of making sense . . . start to develop a script about who you are now. You need a way of demonstrating the kind of behavior that represents the new person you are becoming."[83] Adjusting to a new identity and accepting a new social circle go hand in hand.

Trish Hambridge has worked particularly hard to develop relationships that work in her current condition. She looks for opportunities to socialize with others suffering from aphasia, finding it helpful to connect with those who face similar challenges. It is also an effective way to work on improving her language. She has gone on several vacations organized by the Aphasia Recovery Connection (ARC), which have been particularly rewarding. Her father Doug said, "The whole ARC thing has been a great experience for her in terms of the people involved and the number of activities she's been involved with."

Julia Fox Garrison, a self-proclaimed extrovert by nature, shared the positive outlook on an evolved social life. Realizing that her recovery required a lot of positive energy, she drifted away from her friends who weren't naturally optimistic and became even closer to those who were. "I learned who is my real friend. I thank my stroke for helping me to cut out most of the negativity and negative people in my life." That may seem extreme, but Julia isn't the only one of us who appreciates how her stroke made her rethink her priorities and surroundings.

Said Andrea Helft, "I think stroke has improved me. I do. I think I'm happier and probably healthier—better in a lot of ways. I might even do it again if I had to. Isn't that crazy? I think my relationships are deeper, too. There have been some really big downsides, but overall, I feel like it was a good thing." This level of optimism is pretty uncommon. But it is a testament to the importance of relationships (with or without stroke recovery) and the fact that there really are powerful silver linings for most people going through stroke recovery.

. . .

I've found myself getting even closer to my closest friends. Some of that may relate to my having more time to spend with those who also have the time. Lizzie Bradley, Tony Stayner, and Beth Cross were already among my best friends. So were the members of my long-time support group. All of them have provided me with incredible assistance. They also played a huge role in helping me rediscover my new social identity, and in the process, our relationships have changed. Some of my friends have experienced significant life crises of their own, and I think I've become a more caring and supportive friend to them having gone through this process and changed myself.

It's painful to accept the fact that some friendships will evolve and perhaps grow apart. Many of my professional friends, who were important to me because my career and our shared work and values were so important to me, have definitely drifted away. I don't blame them at all—it's somewhat natural now that I'm no longer engaged in the work that brought us together. And all of us are busy with family, work, and life. It's the natural impact of shifting priorities, changed activities, lessened abilities, and the same amount of time in a year.

There are new friendships as well. Karen Jordan, Steve's classmate who started helping out with Kaya, asked if she and I could just put a weekly walk on the calendar once she found out that walking had become part of my routine. No creativity needed on my part. No request I needed to make. I could just accept, which I did. The offer was particularly touching because I knew how busy she was. For more than a year, we walked almost every week. She's now among my closest friends, independent of her relationship with Steve. Another silver lining.

And of course, many relationships have changed. I stayed with my friend and former colleague Robin Ely and her husband Harry Spence for four months while doing a clinical trial in Boston, and I still talk to her at least once a month on the phone now. We are in some ways closer than ever, intimate and connected as she said. But she also admits that in certain ways, there's a little more distance than there was before. We initially bonded over shared professional values and the work we did together, and can no longer build our relationship on that same foundation. Identity is dynamic and "constantly being confirmed and modified in negotiation with others," wrote Sally Maitlis.[84] Our changing relationship reflects and informs my changing sense of self, as our bond and my identity are now based less on professional work and more on social connection.

PEOPLE ARE SOCIAL ANIMALS: CHAPTER 11 HIGHLIGHTS

- People are fundamentally social by nature; we all need friends and a social life to be happy.
- This can be hard after stroke, and there are real reasons to reduce or avoid socializing.
- But it is critical to overcome these barriers and reestablish a social life, whether with old friends or new ones.
- Social interactions are very important ways for survivors to experiment with and learn about our changing identities.
- Relationships may change, and some may fade, but others may emerge or become stronger than ever.

CHAPTER 12.

How the World Responds

In 2016, six years after my stroke, Steve and I decided it was time for a family adventure. We found a great deal on a trip to Peru, including a four-day trek and a visit to Machu Picchu. Most friends thought we were crazy. I still walked slowly with a limp, had no function of my right arm, and needed significant stretching and warm-ups for daily life. How was I going to complete a four-day trek through the Andes going as high as fifteen thousand feet?

But I'm stubborn, and my family knew that taking a trip like this would have emotional significance for me. The local guide group used pack horses to carry gear on this trek, and Steve confirmed they could bring a saddle horse that I could ride whenever the walking was too much for me or we needed to cover ground faster than I could walk. We spent nearly a week in spectacular mountains, just our family and guides. The only other people we saw were a few locals walking the trail to bring goods to a town market. It was invigorating to be active, relaxing to bond with family, and refreshing to be in such an isolated place. The stars were as bright as I've ever seen. For once, I wasn't trying to fit into the expectations of the world I couldn't keep pace with.

After our mountain trek, along with a few thousand other travelers, we took the bus up to the famous ruins of Machu Picchu. It was gorgeous, inspiring, and crowded. We spent the whole day walking around the ruins. Toward the end of the day, I was walking down some stone steps with my walking stick in my left hand, staying near the wall to stabilize myself. A group of people who were oblivious to my efforts rushed quickly by and made it hard for me to keep my safe position. I think I elbowed one of them, half intentionally, and glared as they went by.

On the next staircase, an older man watched a similar scene developing and, with the best of intentions, reached out a helping hand. I glared at him too, and forcefully waved him away. I had just walked and ridden a horse for four days in the mountains and had been walking around the ruins all day without any problems. "I don't need your help," I made clear through gestures and a glare. Steve caught my arm, afraid that I was about to swing my walking stick at him.

I react that way often. I get angry when people don't respect the needs of people with disabilities, but I also don't want anybody's pity or for them to assume that I can't take care of myself. I certainly don't want their first impression of me to be that something's wrong and I need help. But I do sometimes need help.

Those of us with disabilities, physical or speech or otherwise, find ourselves in a world that is frankly not built or prepared for us. Sometimes we aren't prepared for the reactions in the world around us either. I had to learn that my own actions seem contradictory to others, and that I need to help them understand my own reactions better.

Yes, I have disabilities. No, that does not need to define me. Now I try to be more forceful in asking for help when I need it, and also in asking for the time or patience or other accommodations that I might need to go it alone. I try to do it with more grace than I did on the steps of Machu Picchu, but Steve does still worry that if I sense someone judging me as a person based on my disabilities, they might get a walking stick to the shin.

• • •

What does it mean to have a disability? According to the American Psychological Association (APA), "A disability is a condition or quality linked to a particular person. A disability is present when activities usually performed by people (such as walking, talking, reading, learning) are in some way restricted." Of course, the disabilities vary greatly, nearly 20 percent of the American population, over fifty million people, live with a disability, according to the United States Census.[85] The APA, like others, makes it very clear that "people have disabilities," rather than "a person is disabled," which would suggest that disability categorizes or even defines them.

The world is not oriented toward accommodating those with disabilities, and there is little we can do to avoid a fairly constant barrage of insensitive actions. In *Tempered Radicals*, I discussed psychological armoring, a tactic that people use to defend themselves against threats to their identity and self-esteem.[86] This technique is most often used to offer self-caring to underrepresented minorities in racist encounters. But it can apply in any situation where his or her visible differences make someone feel out of place. We can armor ourselves: create a separation between our internal feeling of self-worth and the external world's treatment of us.

It often takes awhile for stroke survivors to realize the need for strategies like armoring. One study of stroke survivors found, "They were surprised by how interactions with other people changed after the stroke."[87] Those studied found that they were very vulnerable to how others treated them, and that "others could undermine their position" during the interaction, ignoring or talking down to them. This isn't usually intentional but happens in daily interactions. Some of the participants found that they began to de-personalize interactions with others completely. If people treated them as inferior, they began to think of themselves differently, too.

• • •

Cindy Lopez is a vibrant woman with a dazzling smile. A grants manager living in Massachusetts and of Filipino descent, Cindy had a stroke when she was thirty-six. More prepared than most for the recovery process, she already knew how to get past the "why me" stage because her husband had overcome a serious illness about a decade earlier. She was less prepared for living with the ongoing disabilities that stroke has left her with.

"I was thirty-six at the time, and I looked a lot younger than that," she said. Before stroke, she would have walked up to a bar and seen appreciation in people's eyes. Now she walks with a cane, and reactions are much different. "People were always like, 'What happened to you? There's something wrong.'"

Cindy has faced head-on how much of our identity is tied up in our relationship with others and in how they see us. "People in my age group go out a lot trying to meet others, and they are not looking at me thinking, 'Oh, you're so cute,'" she said, which is what she's used to. Instead, "It's like, 'Oh my God—what's wrong with you?' You can actually see the look of disgust in some people's eyes."

One reason for such painful interactions is that visible disabilities often become a master status to able-bodied people, although they probably don't realize that is happening. "Master status is the primary characteristic by which an individual is socially identified."[88] We all look to social cues and patterns to categorize and judge other people. This is not a conscious exercise—it's a subconscious and evolutionary one. That's why it can lead two parties in an interaction to reach such different conclusions.

It was clear to Cindy that she needed help to adapt to the new body she occupied and to how others would respond to her. She looked online for resources and found nothing for younger stroke survivors, despite this being the most pressing issue for her and many other survivors. "In interactions with other people, disability becomes the salient reference. Identity and self-definition are the driving influences in [the stroke survivor's] life," wrote the authors of a study of in *Sociology of Health & Illness*. "Survivors in our research emphasized that being characterized by their stroke impairments made it difficult to reestablish normal relationships with others."[89] Cindy now sees a therapist, spending most of their sessions talking through what it means to adjust to who she is now.

Many people treat those with stroke symptoms as mentally impaired. "I think my biggest issue is people's assumptions about us," said Kathy Howard with a bit of harshness in her voice that reflects the pain this issue brings. Prior to her stroke, Kathy had been in charge of a particular program at her church, and the new committee was planning a meeting to discuss the next year's program. A lady whom Kathy had known for over forty years approached Kathy's husband, Jim, one Sunday after service to explain that they would like Kathy to come to the meeting so that they could pick her brain. Kathy couldn't believe it. She was standing right next to Jim while this conversation was going on; the woman wanted to pick her brain, but she never once looked at Kathy or addressed her directly. "I was crushed," Kathy said. "I've known her for years, and she lives right around the corner from us."

When the same woman approached Jim again the following week, Kathy looked at her and outright told her, "Jim doesn't make my calendar, I do." Kathy regretted that the woman was embarrassed by her response, but at the same time she realized that stroke survivors have a job to do in educating others about stroke because so many people don't understand it. "I've been kind of on a mission since then," Kathy said.

Martina Varnado, who is battling multiple sclerosis, faces similar reactions. "People look at me, they look at the chair, and they draw conclusions," she said. "I may ask a question, then they look to [my husband] Art and give him the answer." Sometimes Art will look away so the person cannot make eye contact with him and must look at Martina directly. Other times, Martina will simply request that they speak with her. She acknowledges that sometimes she gets resentful and addresses people more harshly than she should. She hopes people don't get too offended but also reminds herself that the burden for communicating properly can't only rest with the people with disabilities. She doesn't expect people to ignore the fact that she is in a wheelchair, but the way in which they acknowledge it could be far more thoughtful. Some make jokes, trying to make light of the situation without realizing how offensive that is. Others set a great example. Martina described one contact that she found particularly impressive. "We were at the mall, and Art asked a woman if there was a family bathroom. The woman replied, 'Does one of you need special accommodation, because I can lead you to the right place if so.'" Her lack of presumption that she— in the wheelchair—was not necessarily the one with special needs in this instance was a much-appreciated sign of respect.

When disabilities are less visible, a different set of issues can come into play. Ahaana Singh is thankful that she recovered most of her physical capabilities quickly, but she still has cognitive deficits. She struggles with things she did easily before, and people aren't very patient with her. "Everybody treats me like nothing's happened, and they don't ever ask me how I'm doing," she said. "They think I'm just over it, that I'm completely recovered. But I'm not." She's battling depression already and feels let down by the people she thought she could count on. A disability can still be painful and crippling even if others can't see it on the surface, and Ahaana's frustration at the lack of understanding is evident.

Ahaana often refutes her husband's claim that she is the same person. "I'm not the same person, and I think all stroke survivors have that problem," she said. As stroke survivors go through identity crises and rediscovery, their treatment by others can have major consequences. Identity is in part socially constructed, after all.

Unfortunately, sudden disability can fray relationships and interactions not just with strangers and acquaintances but also with close friends. "You lose all the friends you thought you were close to. It's as if you fell off the face of the earth," said one participant in a large stroke study. "I don't know why, but it's one of the hardest things I had to deal with. I was in the hospital, and I don't think half of my friends came to see me, ever. It's too close to home for them. I mean if it can happen to one person, it might happen to them, and that's scary."[90] While techniques like psychological armoring and conscious attempts to surround yourself with people who understand and adapt to the disability are effective, it's hard to dull the blow of losing close friends or social standing, or to feel fully invulnerable to how others treat you.

. . .

Recently, I expressed hesitancy about reaching out to one close friend, and for the first time explained that I thought this friend felt pity for me. Steve followed up: what is the line between feeling legitimately sorry that you are in this situation (good) and feeling pity for you (bad)? That led to a great family conversation. Among many thoughts on the topic, one really stood out: feeling sorry is about the situation, feeling pity is about the person.

I want people to empathize with my stroke and the challenges I face, but I don't want them to see me and my life as just the stroke and its consequences and to pity me as a result. Yes, recovering from stroke is frustrating and painful and sometimes a nightmare. But my life is not a nightmare—in many ways it is blessed. I want people to think of me for all parts of my identity and life, not just for what I have lost because of my stroke.

Proactively taking control of a situation can help others react in more positive ways. Trish Hambridge was constantly frustrated with how people tried to jump in and help with her speech by guessing at her intent or rushing her, completely insensitive to the challenges of aphasia. She learned that the best way to interact in social settings, especially with strangers, was to come right out and say, "I have a speech disorder," as soon as they met or when a conversation was just starting. She finds that interactions with new people are far more pleasant when they are aware of her disability immediately. Her experience has been that most people really want to create space for her, even if that costs them more time. "It's like they get in touch with their kinder self." Trish likes to think that her approach makes the encounter better for her, and in some small way helps others as well.

I've adopted this strategy since Trish shared it, and I find it extremely helpful with strangers. I tend to be a bit more blunt when people interrupt me or are impatient; I tell them, "Let me talk." A bumper sticker outside a hospital in Boston shares, "Aphasia is loss of communication ability, not intellect." Others will not act differently until those of us most affected help them learn.

In *Tempered Radicals*, I wrote, "One way to wear psychological armor is to channel frustration and rage to avoid being controlled by these emotions." Peter Grant was an African-American whose father taught him the choice was simple: "he could be a victim of racism and be at the mercy of his own anger or he could rise above and try to do something about it."[91] We can't often control how other people react to us, but we can control how we interact with them. We can consciously separate our esteem and identity from their reactions; we can correct and inform them; and perhaps, we can even use our difference to inspire change.

HOW THE WORLD RESPONDS: CHAPTER 12 HIGHLIGHTS

- Unfortunately, the world is often not built well for people with disabilities.
- It can be hard for even well-meaning people to effectively balance a desire to acknowledge and recognize your disability by helping, and not assuming that you are incapable and need help.
- People will make assumptions or treat you differently because of a disability; try not to let this make you angry or impact your view of self-worth.
- Instead, try to create strategies to manage others' reactions and tell them how you would like to be treated.

CHAPTER 13

Activities Adapted

In 2005, when my children were ten, fourteen, and sixteen, we were skiing in Utah at an area we had never skied before. Someone told us there was a great run if we hiked a bit from the top of the main lift then traversed along the ridge just a few minutes further. We made the short trek, and when Adam arrived at the top of the recommended area, he was off. Danny followed right behind. I got there next and looked into a moderate chute—a steep, narrow entry that fed into a more open slope about thirty yards below. By this time, all three kids were pretty strong skiers, but Sarah was only ten. I looked back at Steve and Sarah, who were just behind me, and said something to the effect of, "I know you're skiing well, Sarah, but this may be a bit much." She slid up beside me, looked in, glanced sideways at me, and groaned, "Mooom," and in she went. Several quick turns and she was out the other end.

I looked at Steve, and we didn't even have to say anything. Skiing was our family activity. Steve and I were both strong skiers, and we always said we'd invest the time on beginner slopes to teach the kids well, so we could have a lifetime of skiing together as a family.

Now, on family vacations to the mountains, I'm the one left behind.

• • •

The activities that we fill our time with are one of the purest expressions of what we care about and how we define ourselves. We can't always completely choose our family, friends, relationships, or careers, but our activities and hobbies are selected precisely for how we want to live and who we want to be. To have those taken away from us is a direct affront to the image of ourselves we have deliberately created.

From a young age, I had loved sailing. It was something I did with my parents at first, and for them it was all about having fun. But I quickly became competitive, racing dinghies in Lake St. Clair. Larry Bacow was my sailing instructor at Great Lakes Yacht Club beginning when I was thirteen years old and would become my good friend and mentor. "You were a bundle of energy, fiercely competitive—and the best of the female sailors, by a long way," he remembers. I used to hate it when they split up the girls and the boys for races—I wanted to compete against the whole group, not just half of it.

One day we were sailing on Lake St. Clair and an offshore squall came through and flipped our boat. A Coast Guard helicopter came over, thinking we were in distress, worried the wind would blow us farther out. In truth, we frequently practiced capsize drills, so we knew exactly how to get the boat back up ourselves, but now we couldn't because of the downdraft from the helicopter. At a young age, I was confident, determined, and hated it when people assumed I couldn't do something I believed I could. Sailing was one place I channeled lots of my energy for years, including four years of varsity sailing in college and eventually leading to my family living on a sailboat for a year.

We have all built up a rich set of experiences and passions that define who we are. Losing the ability to continue them is painful. When we are not busy, our minds naturally turn to the things we used to spend our time doing and what we have lost. In *Flow: The Psychology of Optimal Experience*, psychologist Mihály Csíkszentmihályi found that people are happiest when engaged in activities (work or pleasure) that they find stimulating, challenging, and appropriate to their skillset.[92] This happens frequently in music, sports, and other physical activities. Often, for stroke survivors, these activities we loved before are now out of reach. We have built skill sets, social groups, and attitudes around them. A significant piece of our satisfaction in life is built around them. It is hard to move on when they've been taken away.

When I met with Malik Thoma in a café to talk about his experience of stroke, he pulled out a photograph and told me, "My mother wanted me to show you this, so you can see what I used to be." The photo shows a muscular man standing in bright sunlight on the prow of a sailboat at anchor in a harbor of azure water. He looks strong, I tell him. "Yes, I was," he said, putting the photo away and pulling out his resume that detailed his career, community leadership, investing, and sporting activities. As we talked, Malik made it very clear that without the achievements listed on those pages, the person he used to be is gone. His physical disabilities now prevent him from doing many of them, involving both work and play. However, rather than finding new activities that give him pleasure and meaning, Malik is, unfortunately and painfully, still focused primarily on what he has lost.

Intentional sensemaking can help stroke survivors move past the initial trauma and deficits. Instead of mourning the loss of an activity forever, we can analyze the reasons why it was so important and search for new ways to fill that need. Maitlis describes the process that I went through, and wish I had understood earlier:

> *In the struggle to come to terms with the new reality that follows a trauma, people are forced to give up certain assumptions and goals and to work to create new meanings and a new understanding of the world and of themselves in that world. This process is both confusing and painful but contains the opportunity for significant change. During these times, people notice new things and perceive old things in different ways, often provoking insights that enable different ways of being.[93]*

Athleticism and a life of physical activity have always been central to my mental picture of myself. I used to cherish my almost daily jog—early in my recovery, I pushed hard to return to running. My therapists had to slow me down on the treadmill; even walking fast, let alone jogging, would hurt my form and work against my rehab efforts. I do miss running, but years later, it's not nearly as important as it was. I have found ways to replace my run with a mix of other activities that get my heart rate up (walking hills), give me solitude (swimming), and hold on to my identity as an athlete (tandem biking). I might not be able to sail or bike like I used to, but I still find value and enjoy being a sailing instructor to my kids and taking tandem bike rides with Steve. It's been really important for me to really think about the lost activities and develop insights into why they were valuable in the first place. "These insights can provide individuals with the opportunity to rework and reassemble their experiences, and thus to reinvent themselves," wrote Maitlis.

· · ·

I first met Anthony Santos in the reception area of the therapy center we both attend. Anthony was a healthy young man ready to launch into his chosen career as a nurse when he had a stroke following a standard surgical procedure. Previously an active, athletic boy, he now had no significant control of his left leg and arm, and he was confined to a wheelchair. He was nineteen.

When I asked about her son's recovery process, Anthony's mother Martina quickly mentions sports, "Before, sports gave him a lot of pleasure. For the first few months after the stroke, he had almost no pleasure at all because he wasn't making any progress and couldn't play any sports." Like my kids at his age, Anthony's life revolved around baseball, snowboarding, wakeboarding, hiking, riding motorcycles, and more.

Initially wheelchair bound, his ability to walk and grasp objects improves daily, even three years after his stroke. "When I was in the wheelchair, and I couldn't do anything at all, my confidence was low just because I couldn't do anything that I was previously able to do. Now, as I'm doing more things, as I'm walking independently, it's slowly rising up. As I continue to get even better, it will continue to rise up." Anthony is very clear that being an independently active man is a big part of his determination in rehab. But he's still got a way to go before he reclaims the activities he loved.

"I'm impatient and . . . scared, I guess you could say," said Anthony. "I don't know what my future looks like. I mean, I would love for it to head forward, but there's no guarantee that I'm gonna get better." Still in his early twenties, Anthony has no thought of giving up his goals and progress. He continues to focus on small wins, new activities, and battling hard for continued progress. His determination and positive outlook have yielded exciting progress already in the fifteen months between our two conversations. Before, he could barely walk five hundred feet before getting tired. Now, he had just returned from Mexico and had enjoyed touring around, walking, and appreciating the vacation. This has all come about after the typical twelve-month recovery cutoff so often promoted by the medical system. "I never believed there could be no progress after twelve months. Now that I've found the right therapy, it's obviously not true," Anthony said.

He's doing lots of hiking now, and he is focused on wakeboarding as the first among his previous sports to try again because it requires less fine motor control. Martina joined the conversation in Spanish (with Anthony translating for us). "This is true. Just last weekend you went out to play tennis and that was the happiest I've seen you since the stroke." He also went to a beach and was walking around, climbing dunes that lead down to the shore, and his mother could just see in his face how happy he was.

· · ·

Adapting to new activities sometimes feels inadequate. I appreciate and even savor my tandem bike rides with Steve, but I can't pretend the reliance on his schedule, the view of his back, or the constant tinkering to make various braces and angles work isn't a step down from solo riding. I give myself room for that occasional "pity party," but mostly I celebrate that we have found a way for me to keep riding a regular part of my life. We have made it the foundation for several great cycling vacations.

Trish Hambridge used to play softball and soccer, and according to her friend Delia, she feels that loss. But she's found a group of stroke survivors who all play golf together, and she now relishes that. Just as Steve and I have had to tinker endlessly to make our tandem bike work well, Trish's dad has worked on her golf clubs to make them usable. "He kind of MacGuyver-ed a club so that she could work it," said Delia. Along with golf for the athletic piece, Trish now walks constantly for exercise. She still misses softball and soccer, of course, but she's found new physical activities that are sources of enjoyment.

Activities may now require trade-offs that I never considered before. I missed skiing desperately, and when I felt ready to tackle a beginner slope again, my physical therapist warned me against it. She was worried the pressure, rigid boot, and risk of injury would jeopardize my rehab progress. I'm still working to walk in proper form, after all. But in this case, I decided some risk was worth the joy of skiing again. I don't do it as often as I might otherwise, and I am very cautious. I've learned that as important as physical rehab is, it's only part of recovery—we are working to rebuild our entire lives.

As I think about my activities now and pre-stroke, it feels as if the packaging is different, but the underlying values and goals remain pretty much the same. By thinking deeply about what matters, rather than just discarding those critically important pieces of our identity embodied in our activities, we can adapt and find new ways to enjoy them.

A vital part of the rebuilding process has been acknowledging, if not celebrating, my identity as a stroke survivor. I now work with the Pacific

Stroke Association to help others to thrive after stroke. By embracing my stroke—and writing this book—I am also able to achieve the thing I have always loved most in my professional life: to explore and generate knowledge, to teach, and to make a difference in the world. Says Maitlis, "Positive identity can be understood as a central element of a growth story."[94]

A cross-country bike trip had always been on the bucket list for Steve and me. It was one of many items on a wish list that tended to accumulate goals faster than achieving them. Now, it has taken on major meaning that combines many of the activities and values I care most about: we've set a goal to do a family cross-country ride sometime after this book is released—to raise money and awareness for stroke prevention and rehabilitation.

ACTIVITIES ADAPTED: CHAPTER 13 HIGHLIGHTS

- Very often, our favorite activities will be out of reach after a stroke.
- This is particularly painful as activities are often our purest expression of what we enjoy, and we have built relationships, skills, and lives around them.
- Some can be reclaimed after improvements gained through the hard work of therapy.
- And for those we can't reclaim, if we understand why we cared about an activity, we can often adapt a previous activity or find new ones to get much of the same pleasure.

CHAPTER 14.

Careers and Callings

On YouTube, there is a video of a lecture I gave at Stanford in November 2005, five years before my stroke. As I watch that video now, I am struck by how different that Debra is from the Debra of today. The Debra in the video speaks quickly, with assurance and authority. Her hand gestures are light and fluid. The timbre of her voice is higher than mine now—not unpleasantly high but with a pitch that seems driven by energy.

This version of Debra was the "me" that I compared myself with in those early months after my stroke. I was Debra Meyerson the professor, the speaker, teacher, and creator of knowledge. I was an independent woman, who had balanced family and career success in a field I cared deeply about. Except that I wasn't anymore.

The grief I felt when that identity was officially taken away from me was overwhelming. The bond between my work and my sense of self was so tight that I barely even questioned *why* work was so important; it just seemed obvious. Conversely, my inability to work in the way that I wanted led to a crisis of self-doubt.

About three years after my stroke, I started asking myself more deliberately why I cared so much, and what values drove me to do what I did. Many other survivors I had talked to felt similarly about their lost careers, but certainly not all. I felt that understanding what I cared most about would help me continue on my recovery with more motivation and direction. Family was most important. After that was my work as a professor; more than a job, my vocation was a calling. I realized that to me, my Stanford professorship actually represented every level of Maslow's pyramid: security (paycheck), esteem and belonging (validated work and colleagues), and fulfillment and actualization through meaningful work in diversity and gender issues.

Losing this much was a blow, and parts can never be recovered. But understanding what lay underneath my attachment to career let me begin to replace it, or at least rebuild each section more intentionally.

· · ·

"One's work is believed to provide one with many things," wrote Mike Pratt and Blake Ashforth in *Positive Organizational Scholarship*, "economic gain, social status, a sense of belonging, and even a sense of purpose or meaning."[95] For many stroke survivors, these are all taken away at once. Consuming the bulk of our waking hours (for many of us), the removal of work leaves a gaping hole in our lives and selves—even if therapy sometimes feels like a full-time job. Work and career play very different roles for different people. For some, work is a job that provides for the basic needs of the family. For others, it may be a critical source of esteem, accomplishment, and meaning. And for some, it's the result of a long commitment and tremendous effort to live out internal values.

Nearly one-third of all stroke survivors are under the age of sixty-five, according to the National Stroke Association. That's approximately 250,000 people each year just in the United States. Of those, probably about 50 percent are unable to return to work, and half of those who do require modifications in the workplace.[96] Those who do return to work after stroke may struggle with various obstacles like self-consciousness, negative reactions from colleagues or clients, and unexpected fatigue.

This is a problem that is growing: stroke incidence in younger adulthood is increasing, and working past sixty-five is becoming more common due to longer life expectancy and financial need.[97] A study of changing identity after aphasic stroke noted, "Participants spoke about the difficulty they had accepting this and their struggle to find some kind of work they could do."[98] Work in today's society is not just a means to pay bills; it is often a core part of our identity.

That produces some interesting dynamics in the way our careers fit into our lives, and they are different from those of past generations. "Paradoxically, the 'working class' is spending fewer hours at work, while the erstwhile 'leisure class' has less leisure," found *Time for Life*, an analysis of how people spend their time. "Whether this implicit trade-off in the distribution of time and money is psychologically or morally satisfying for either group is a perplexing question."[99] One natural conclusion is this: as we climb Maslow's pyramid, the role of work in our lives climbs with us. It does not have a single meaning but rather a dynamic one, just like our identities.

. . .

Manny Gigante has managed to work past his disappointments and look to the future. He was an unapologetic type-A personality before his stroke, with a good career as a network engineer. Fit and active as a twenty-nine-year-old, he would climb towers, fix wires, and ride a motorcycle, moving fast with big goals and prospects. "I will be the first to admit that if there was a dollar sign attached to something, that's what I was drawn to," he said. "I had this idea implanted in my head that the way you become successful in life is to work as hard as you can and make as much money as you can."

He had built his life and his family around this view of success and a good life. He knew that his family had certain expectations that he should fulfill. "Coming from my Filipino cultural background, you don't share weaknesses." His role was to be the breadwinner, teach his kid to play sports, and set an example of strength and dependability. He pursued that vision without much thought about the meaning behind it. "I never took the time to even think of a five-year plan," he said, reflecting that in some ways his pursuit of success was about his immediate needs, not truly about family. "You're not supposed to be vulnerable," he said.

After his stroke, he struggled with the sudden gaps in his abilities. "I took the victim role; I took the shame role," he said. He had invested so much in his vision of himself and his career. He had built his life around those images. Early on after the stroke, he was single-mindedly dedicated to recovering everything. He would get back his job as an engineer; he'd get everything back. "Oh, I'm going to get back to 100 percent and be able to ride a motorcycle again."

But the progress was slow. He was in a wheelchair for the first two years, forced to reconcile a vision of himself with a very different reality. His situation is common for younger stroke survivors. In one study of young stroke survivors, every participant believed that the process of returning to work was a critical and valuable goal. One of them said, "The thought process inside my head was, 'Disability is other people and disability isn't me. I'm not disabled and I'm not going to be disabled.'"[100] Yet each had to come to grips with a new reality. Said Manny, "It's been a struggle for me to overcome my disability and rewire my brain to think another way."

Over time, Manny realized that his old job was too physical, but that was OK. "I came to finally accept that I couldn't dream to be back to where I was 100 percent," he said. He began to set his sights not on the past but on the future. "Any improvement is a victory in and of itself, and I've been able to accept that as progress . . . I'm able to celebrate the small victories." Manny adopted the practice of focusing on small wins, which added up to big progress over time, and had a far more positive attitude about his situation.

He started with his own family: work was, before anything else, about providing for himself and them—the bottom of Maslow's pyramid.

"Basically, I had to redesign my life around my new reality and resign myself to the fact that it wasn't just about me anymore." Instead of seeking the kind of high-flying job he had before, he looked for something less physical that gave him a paycheck and more time with his family at home. At the time, real estate was hot in the Bay Area, so he got involved in that.

He also changed his entire approach to work. "My occupation is mortgage consultant, a loan officer, and basically, the hierarchy started at the top with an attorney, then there was a used car salesman, then the garbage man, and then the loan officer. There was such a stigma attached to the job." But he was no longer in it for the reputation or himself. In reevaluating his priorities, it wasn't just that he wanted to support his family; he had found a deeper meaning. "It was about how could I help as many families as I could. Once I took that approach, my life was changed forever."

Whereas people in the job before him were "just out to get money," he said he's changed the process. He wants to educate his customers and make it his first priority to help them get into the house they want for less money long-term—to save them money. "It's a huge shift. For a long time, it was just gimme, gimme, gimme for me. How can Manny make the most out of each deal," he remembered of his previous life. "Now I'm taking a step back and finding the more people I serve in that way, the better I feel. It's deeply satisfying." And he actually finds that his altered attitude comes back to him in the form of a great reputation, good referrals, and more business.

Manny's stroke changed his conception of a successful life and career— before, they were the same. "I learned to be more patient and to understand what's really important in life. I accepted the reality of where I am now. I've heard so many people say, 'If only I had blank, I could be blank.' Having my disability, I've realized that's not the case. As long as I am breathing, then I can do whatever I want." For Manny, doing whatever he wants has a new meaning. It's not about a specific job; it's about finding a way to live out his true values.

Manny also sees that his evolution has started to reshape the way his family values work. "Being part of an immigrant family in America, my parents' dream was, 'You gotta go to college. You gotta have a job with a good, stable company,'" and he pursued that goal. But now he sees that "It's passion that gets you where you want to go." He discovered that if he identified the things he really cared about, he could work around his disability and find ways to pursue new goals. That may bother his more traditional mother, but it has inspired his daughter. "My oldest daughter has actually decided to become an occupational therapist because of her experience with me," said Manny. "That just filled my heart. I am, like, wow. I see the compassion in my daughter that grew out from me. I thought I would be a hindrance in her life, but I am actually shaping it."

. . .

Many stroke survivors who loved their previous career struggle to let it go and look forward. One former professional who was left with severe aphasia described how he repeatedly drove to his office and tried to engage in his old job, ultimately unsuccessfully.[101] Teresa, a professional mezzo-soprano who lost her ability to sing after cancer, worked hard to regain her voice but was beset with failure. Finally, she conceded defeat: "I just couldn't handle that, you know? Then I was leaning on the piano in the studio, and [my teacher] was sitting at the keyboard. We were having a very sad lesson . . . and he looked at me and said, 'Why don't you just stop coming?' And I said, 'You're right.' And that's the last time I went to the studio."[102]

Six years after his stroke, Malik Thoma still feels as if it stole a core piece of his identity that is simply irreplaceable. He worked constantly to run his chain of day spas and loved what he did. He invested himself fully in it, and his work was also a massive source of stress. Malik's wife thinks it's one of the reasons he had his stroke. After the stroke, he tried to return to work and find other jobs but was unable to. "Every two hours, I would be mentally exhausted and have to stop and not do anything for a while. It was just excruciating. I was going at one-tenth the pace I had in the past." The comparison with his past life and capabilities makes it hard for Malik to find satisfaction in accomplishments now. "I've taught my kids their multiplication tables and things like that," he said when thinking about accomplishments. "But that's not really something you can point to as a good accomplishment."

Unlike Manny, Malik has not been able to look forward and leverage small wins. The difference that healthy goal setting can make to this kind of situation is massive. "By itself, one small win may seem unimportant. A series of wins at small but significant tasks, however, reveals a pattern that may attract allies, deter opponents, and lower resistance to subsequent proposals," said Professor Karl Weick. "Small wins are controllable opportunities that produce visible results."[103] Being able to see accomplishments, even if they are small, could put Malik on a path to improvement.

Sally Maitlis studied professional musicians after stroke as exemplars of those who see work as a calling. She found that, "for anyone whose occupation provides a master status—a role around which other identities are organized—a trauma that prevents them from doing their work is likely to have a significant effect on their self-understanding. Typically, these individuals see their profession not simply as what they do, but as who they are."[104]

Maitlis explored the process as they overcame the loss of their calling. "Each individual now focuses on the core of what matters most to him or her." Since they all had built careers in music, they all had a similar experience of loss. But their paths after stroke varied dramatically as they discovered what it was about music that had mattered so much to them. One loved making music and no longer could do it, so he took to teaching it; one sought a completely different outlet to express newly awakening ideas; one enjoyed the newfound freedom to spend more time with family.

They found positive learning in the experience, and "in the process of constructing these new identities, the musicians began to separate and disassociate from their former selves."[105]

• • •

Julia Fox Garrison was a manager at a software company. Not long into our interview, she said, "I loved my job. I was extremely motivated and driven by it. I was climbing the corporate ladder." Immediately after her stroke, she defaulted to healthy denial and focused on recovery. Julia's stroke meant there were many things she could no longer do, but returning to work was the main focus. "I was going to run again; I was going to get my life back. I tried to go back to work, and it was a disaster."

For Julia, work was far more than a paycheck. Her life was oriented around her job in many ways. "My work life was my social life. Most of my best friends are from my work life. In fact, I met my husband at the last job I had prior to my stroke." As the role of work expands, so does its meaning in our lives. Career is no longer just a way to get a paycheck and secure lifestyle.[106] Julia also had a sense of belonging with her colleagues, and that was a core part of her identity. "I went through a period where I didn't know what I was because I couldn't work anymore," she said.

The lack of meaning in her life after she lost her job and the unintended independence sparked Julia's identity crisis, as well as an examination of what really mattered to her. In a survivor story on this book's website, she wrote, "I could no longer climb the metaphorical corporate ladder. In fact, I couldn't climb anything. I had to relearn everything." And she has. Rather than return to her previous job, she has found a new one that reflects her rebuilt identity as a writer and advocate. She first wrote *Don't Leave Me This Way*, which chronicles her struggle to regain control over her life and body and to deal with the medical system when she was rehabilitating.[107] "I love that I have opportunities to spread my message and hopefully inspire others to think in a positive manner," she said. She makes presentations to health-care professionals, business executives, and other groups to educate and inspire. "My book even won the Applied Association of Therapeutic Humor (AATH) award for furthering their mission—humor in medicine."

Kathy Howard also lost her job after her stroke, but she believes that was a blessing. "Before my stroke, I had some exciting jobs," she said. "I worked for the Department of Justice; I was also a school teacher. But I was always looking." Like so many others, her stroke forced her to work hard to reenter the workplace and to think hard about what kind of job was appropriate for her goals and values. Reflecting on her experience and discovering the lack of emotional resources for survivors, she started Coffee Cafe-sia, for people with aphasia. It started simply, but soon many others joined the dialogue. The group has grown significantly, and Kathy has expanded her work. She wants to help others change their attitudes about stroke, a problem she struggled with herself. "I am on a mission, and I'm working on it all the time. For me, that's very rewarding." She eventually wants to create a therapeutic center where people can come to job hunt, sit and talk with other survivors, or work on rehab together. "I actually have found my dream job," she said. "It was like I kept looking for something, I had a stroke, and now I've found it. In hindsight, maybe having a stroke wasn't the worst thing that ever happened to me."

Julia went even further in her appreciation. "My stroke became a gift to me. It allowed me to do things I never would have been able to do pre-stroke." She embraced the changes far faster than most of us and can look back on the clear difference it made in how she thinks about herself and success. "The pre-stroke Julia had it all together. She was quite successful, and she had achieved the American dream. For poststroke Julia, the success is different. I didn't want to write a book to be famous. I wanted to help people as much as I could, and that was my motivation for writing it. I think the pre-stroke Julia would have been looking for fame."

• • •

Six months after my stroke, I received an invitation from Deborah Stipek, Dean of the School of Education at Stanford, to join her and all the other associate professors for a dinner where we could both build community and discuss the professional path for those with tenured positions seeking promotion to full professorship—the next step up the organizational ladder in academia. At that point, I could barely initiate words, let alone coherent sentences. I felt a sense of vertigo, thinking, "My world continues on, but without me in it!" Eventually, of course, I had to give up my tenure and accept that the career by which I had defined myself was gone.

I also felt that teaching was akin to a calling, and that is perhaps the loss I continue to struggle with most. I may face the frustration every day, but I can also see some of the benefits of my situation since I've crafted a new identity beyond that of *Professor* Debra Meyerson. That role wasn't just about teaching and sharing knowledge; it involved working with doctoral students, researching, university politics, and running a campus center—all sources of much stress. Colleague and friend Robin Ely reminds me that I was constantly stressed before.

I had not been forced to reflect and make choices about what really mattered before my stroke, so I tried to do it all. "I think, you know, she just ran herself ragged," Robin said. "That was what her life was like. That's the kind of thing that she would do." Stress was a constant in my life, and we suspect it played a role in my stroke. Although now I am more frustrated than ever, without all the work-related stress, my tunnel vision is reduced, and I can think about myself in a more balanced, rounded, intentional way. In her study of musicians, Maitlis observed a similar journey as they discovered new aspects of themselves. "I'm not necessarily 'that horn player,'" said one of them. "It has allowed me to move to a better mental idea of what I am and who I am."

More than a decade ago, I wrote in my first book, "Though tempered radicals stay anchored to their core commitments, they must also *remain flexible* about how and when to fulfill them." As I grieved the loss of my author and professor self, I had to confront that reality myself. Successful tempered radicals know who they are and *what is important* to their sense of self. They realize that they have multiple aspects—perhaps even multiple selves. They also realize that some of those aspects are weightier and more important than others, and that sometimes they must adjust how they live out those values.

I had to reflect on *why* I cared so much about being a professor, which I had always taken as a given before my stroke. I found that I missed the students and collegial atmosphere, so I began to observe some classes and advise students where I could. I missed the relationships and sense of belonging. I couldn't get that back in full, but opening myself back up to colleagues put me back in touch with the values and work and discussions that I cared about. And I cared about creating and sharing knowledge, so I began the path that led me to writing this book.[108]

CAREERS AND CALLINGS: CHAPTER 14 HIGHLIGHTS

- Career is important to nearly everyone of working age, though reasons differ. Losing this can be one of the biggest blows from a stroke.

- For some, a career is mostly about financial stability (foundation of Maslow's pyramid), and for others, it is more about meaning and fulfillment (top). For most, it is at least some of both.

- Many working-age survivors can never return to their previous professions.

- It's important to understand what drove you to do the work and if there is another kind of work that can create similar fulfillment.

- For some people, a stroke can prompt self-discovery that leads to a more fulfilling calling post stroke, even with the constraints of disabilities.

CHAPTER 15.

Dealing with Financial Strain

C am Compton lives in St. Louis and was fifty-two when she had a stroke in 2012. She was a medical secretary at Mercy Medical Center where she had worked for thirty years. Divorced a year before her stroke, she was caring for her younger daughter, sixteen at the time, and also her ten-year-old granddaughter. She left the rehab hospital needing to use a walker, and while she ditched it about three months later, she still walks with a limp, has significant weakness in one arm, and has some balance issues. "Sometimes I'm like a drunken sailor on a Friday night," she joked, explaining that all of a sudden, she'll bump into walls, using them to balance and stay upright. She also has stamina issues and what she calls intermittent brain fog.

Before her stroke, Cam's financial situation was comfortably stable. She had a good job with benefits and was making it work to raise two kids, make payments on a modest home, and live a comfortable life. That changed after her stroke. She was unable to work at all for about six months. She eased back in after that, fortunate to have an employer willing to be flexible and work with her to figure out what and how much she could do. She started with two days, four hours each, and eventually worked her way back to twenty-four hours a week and coverage for benefits. At this point, that's all she can handle.

Cam knows she was lucky to have good health insurance, but even with that, her share of the main hospital bill alone was around $20,000, more than she could pay at the time. Lost income had an even bigger impact. Even with good insurance that included short- and long-term disability coverage, she has never regained more than 60 percent of her pre-stroke income. "It was really tough," she said, "especially at the beginning." Her parents and other family helped out a little, but there wasn't much they could do. Bills piled up; some services got cut off. She cut back expenses as best she could: no new clothes, no trips. "I just watched every penny to save where I could."

Cam also got creative and learned there are ways to get help if you ask for it. The biggest problem was that $20,000 hospital bill. "I talk about that one all the time in the stroke support groups I lead," she said. "I told them I just couldn't pay, and I found out they can write off part of the bill if you really have financial hardship. In the end, I paid about half of it."

She also discovered that a lot of people will help if they know you're doing your best. She really didn't want her two girls to suffer because of the financial stress. Her daughter was taking horseback riding lessons, and the center let them pay by having her work in the barn. Another sports program waived the normal fees until Cam got their financial situation a bit more stable.

Cam worked to keep a positive, problem-solving attitude. "Yeah, it was tough to be under such financial stress all of a sudden," she explained. "Sometimes I would get pissed off." But she never let it keep her down; she always looked forward and made the best of it. "I'm not sure," she wondered in our most recent call, acknowledging the irony, "but maybe my brain injury helped me stay positive. When I get stressed, I just have to sleep. And when I wake up, I've usually forgotten what I was stressed or angry about. So I don't hang on to it."

. . .

As in Cam's situation, strokes usually hit financially in two ways. First, it can directly cost survivors and their families a lot of money. An estimate included in a 2014 pamphlet produced by the American Stroke Association called *Finances After Stroke Guide* estimates the lifetime cost of an ischemic stroke at $140,048, including inpatient services, rehab, and follow-up care.[109]

The median family net worth in the United States (50 percent of families have more and 50 percent have less) is $45,000, so that amounts to more than three times their total net worth, most of which is not in savings that can easily be used.[110]

That number is an average. Many strokes are minor, with far fewer associated costs. If you suffer a severe stroke, especially one with a lot of medical complications, the direct hospital costs, even after insurance-negotiated discounts, can be ten times more. The number also doesn't include significant expenses that more affluent survivors incur on their own, outside the insurance system and therefore not tracked in the data. Even more problematic, it is lower than it should be because many survivors stop seeking treatment when insurance stops paying, even if benefits from rehab are still clearly accruing.

For many people, most of the costs will be covered by insurance, but there are deductibles, co-pays, and services that aren't covered. Even after significant increases in enrollment after the Affordable Care Act, 8.8 percent of Americans still didn't have health insurance.[111] People in this situation have far less savings than the average family.

The second economic challenge is lost wages, which for many survivors is even more significant than direct medical costs. More than a quarter of all strokes in the United States are suffered by people sixty-five or under. For those who suffer a more severe event, the inability to work can be financially devastating.

• • •

Randy Miller and his wife Rose were quite comfortable before Randy's stroke at fifty-one. They owned a nice home, were putting their two kids through college, and were on their way toward building savings for retirement fifteen to twenty years out. Now they have had to reorganize life around Randy's ongoing disabilities. The most important is his significant speech challenges from aphasia, but their new financial reality is a big factor, too.

After the stroke, Rose left her job in an orthopedist's office so she could better support Randy, who has not been able to go back to work himself. So, Rose lost her entire salary, and Randy, extremely lucky to have had disability insurance as part of his employee benefits, receives 60 percent of his prior salary. In total, they make less than half of what they did before. "Randy was the major breadwinner," Rose explained. "Now he needs full-time care. On my earnings after tax, I couldn't cover the cost of care, so it made sense for me to leave my job and be the full-time caregiver." This situation is common among survivors and their families.

Even with good medical insurance, their share of the early medical bills for deductibles and co-payments were enough to deplete their savings. Randy was still getting some therapy covered by his insurance three years after his stroke, but it was very limited, so they paid out of pocket for more. When we first met, they were making the tough decision to pay for a speech program at nearby Fontbonne University. They knew it was making a real difference, and Randy so badly wants to regain more functional speech. "I'm always searching for new treatments, new opportunities, things that aren't available with insurance," Rose explained. "But it costs money, you know?"

College loans for their children presented them with more complexity. The good news is they learned that with Randy's disability, they could apply for relief from the fairly significant student loans that funded college for their two kids. They've done so, but are now in a holding period. Payments have been suspended, but a final decision won't be made until they see if Randy is still unable to work in a few more years. Right now, if the loans were discharged, they would have to declare the amount forgiven as income and pay taxes on it. They believe there is a possibility that the law might change, adding uncertainty.

Randy and Rose consider themselves fortunate to have more resources than many to invest in Randy's recovery beyond what insurance will cover. But it has still forced them to make hard choices. They've focused on trimming expenses. They sold a car and trimmed cell phone and cable packages. "We budget more closely than we used to," Rose explained. They used to help out family members with financial needs from time to time, and they supported several foundations for children. Now that's not possible. Some changes have been emotionally difficult. "Before the stroke, we were able to help out our kids as they got started in their adult lives," she said. "We'd buy them small gifts 'just because.' Now I have to think about it more. I got such joy from doing that—it hurts." Their new reality has challenged the aspect of their old identity that related to what it meant to be a good parent.

Trends suggest this is a problem that is only getting more common. A 2016 study found that strokes more than doubled in people ages thirty-five to thirty-nine between 1995 and 2014 and rose in groups up to age fifty-five.[112] The cause is not clear, and with strokes affecting more people in the heart of their working years, this will become an even bigger problem in the future.[113]

Almost every stroke survivor I've met has stories about how life is changing because of financial pressure, from minor to dramatic. Trish Hambridge left her home and friends in California so she could live less expensively in Florida. Michael McDermott lost his job and had to reduce his spending to live on social security. These situations are all very challenging, for sure—and this group of survivors that I interviewed is, on average, more financially stable than most.

Many survivors are struggling to put food on the table because of their strokes. There are those in even more dire straits who were struggling financially before their strokes, and now they have a massive additional burden. A November 2017 article in the *New York Times* told Holly Gambal's story: she had been homeless and living in New York City's subway system for several weeks when she suffered a stroke. Like too many people in America, she suffered from a significant mental illness, fell through the cracks of our medical system, and ended up living on the streets.

• • •

Studying the impact of a trauma like stroke shines a spotlight on the disproportionate disruption born by those with fewer financial resources. Everyone suffers, but some people suffer more. Unfortunately, the disparity is getting worse, because the income and wealth gap in our country is growing. The share of total wealth owned by just the top 1 percent of earners in America has risen from about 9 percent in 1980 to 22 percent in 2013. Over that same period, the average income of the top earners has grown more than four times faster than that of 80 percent of the population. Real wages (wages after accounting for inflation) have grown by 33 percent for the top group; they are up less than 10 percent for people in the middle, and they are actually down for the bottom 10 percent.[114] The racial wealth gap is growing, too. In 2001, the median household wealth for a white family was six times that of the median for black families. By 2013, that number had more than doubled to thirteen times.

Until we can reverse these trends, the financial impact of stroke or any major health crisis will continue to be particularly devastating to our lower-income neighbors and families of color. Unfortunately, the widening financial gap in our society is accompanied by cultural and societal gaps as well. Political polarization is one commonly cited arena, but people are increasingly unlikely to mix with others from different cultural, religious, socio-economic, or other backgrounds and interests. This makes it harder to understand and empathize with others; thus, it becomes harder to fix entrenched problems like income inequality.

The survivors in this book come from a range of backgrounds, but for me it is an uncomfortable reality that most of the survivors I've gotten to know come from backgrounds that are similar to mine—professional, financially comfortable, and focused on seeking great medical care rather than basic needs. I am definitely among the lucky ones. Steve and I both had economically successful careers and were fortunate to have created retirement savings before I suffered my stroke at fifty-three. We were both raised by Depression-era parents who drove home the need to always spend less than you make, no matter how large or small the number. My medical insurance has been good throughout the ordeal, and my benefits with Stanford included a long-term disability policy that, like Randy's, has continued to pay 60 percent of my prior salary. Because I had great support from others, most notably my mom, Steve was able to go back to work fairly quickly.

So, we have had more financial resources than most, which creates huge advantages in navigating the recovery journey. Paying our deductibles didn't strain our economic lives, so that didn't add more stress to an already difficult situation. We could afford to pay for some therapies that insurance didn't cover, which helped my psychological state immensely, since I wanted to do everything possible to advance my recovery. We could purchase assistive devices that were recommended, even when insurance denied coverage.

I'm aware that I have advantages that may make my journey far different than many survivors. Losing my job hurt me emotionally far more than financially. We each struggle with different aspects of our recovery, and finances will play a role in defining our experience, just like other aspects of our unique situations. This is not just about my journey or those of the other survivors in this book; it's about the lessons we can learn from each other in preparing to rebuild life after stroke.

When we first talked a few years ago, Rose told me, "Stroke absolutely stole our future. Our whole life was flipped upside down." When we spoke again two years later, I asked about this issue. They had talked so positively about Randy's progress and how they were active in the community, it didn't seem to fit. "It's a timing thing," she explained in our more recent conversation. "During that first year or two, we were a bit in shock. You make plans for how long you want to work, when you're going to retire, and what you want to do when you retire. You have plans. When Randy had his stroke, our plans were stolen. We didn't get to choose to retire; that choice was made for us. It changed our lifestyle." But now they're making new plans and remind themselves frequently about what they call a new platform for their journey: "Always have hope; never give up."

DEALING WITH FINANCIAL STRAIN:
CHAPTER 15 HIGHLIGHTS

- Financial strain is severe for many survivors, both from medical costs and lost income.

- There are resources available to help, and others will often help if they know you are doing all you can; unfortunately, it's not easy, but research and persistence can really help.

- Insurance is often inadequate, and insurance coverage is still lacking for many; our system really needs comprehensive reform.

- And stroke is clearly harder on those with fewer resources; this will continue to get worse until we find ways to reverse the growing inequality in our society.

CHAPTER 16.

Advocating in the U.S. Medical System

During my first stay in the ICU at Stanford Hospital, Steve came into my room one morning and knew immediately that I was incredibly anxious. At that point, I was mute and not yet very good at communicating in other ways. I was trying to communicate, and he tried to understand, but we quickly realized it was futile. About fifteen minutes later, the nurse assigned to my room returned to take some vital signs and replenish an IV drip. She started talking to me in the same tone I had been enduring since her shift began earlier that morning: a high-pitched, syrupy, slow, and overly enunciated voice that is so often used when adults talk to infants. I don't know why, but a small minority of caregivers think that voice is sweet and caring. I think that if infants could talk, they, like me, would say it's condescending and obnoxious.

When she finished her tasks and started out of the room, I screwed my face into a lopsided grimace, bared my teeth, and shook my left fist at her back as she departed. I didn't have to speak; Steve now knew precisely why I was agitated. He calmed me down and said he'd see what he could do. He tracked the nurse down in an unoccupied part of the corridor and explained to her that I was anxious; that her tone was upsetting me; and that her normal voice in a straightforward conversation, with longer pauses to wait for a reaction due to my aphasia, would be much more effective with me and very much appreciated. She was clearly a bit put off, but she tried to be gracious and accepted his request. Unfortunately, her next trip into the room was little different from the last, and my fist was flying again when she left.

Steve is generally reluctant to tell someone else how to run their operation, but after a few more attempts to influence the nurse's approach with no success, he found the ICU nursing supervisor. Explaining that this nurse was not helping my condition, he asked that they assign someone else to my room in the future. The staff made sure I had other nurses during my stay in the ICU, and it was far less stressful thereafter. This episode convinced Steve that he (and others on my team) had to be my constant advocates. And as my condition improved, I had to be my own advocate.

Overall, the care I received at Stanford was exceptional. But it is a large hospital with hundreds of staff and thousands of patients, all in a very high-stress environment. Nobody could be as attuned to my needs and desires in my recovery process as we were. We learned that where we had issues or questions, we should voice them. We have found that most people are highly receptive and even eager to improve care. Most of our questions just led to clarification and explanation because nothing was wrong. But in a time of so much uncertainty, confusion and anxiety, that too was helpful. And periodically our questions actually did change the nature and quality of my care.

The American medical system has become a huge industrial complex that can't always deliver what is best for the individual needing care. So, we learned to look out and advocate for ourselves. This was true in the ICU, in choosing hospitals and therapy programs, in finding and negotiating for more therapy options, and in battling insurance companies to get coverage. The hospitals we used are great institutions. Almost all of our doctors, nurses, therapists, and other caregivers were caring, committed, and skilled. But we still found it critical to fully own the responsibility for getting what we thought I needed, pushing beyond the temptation to trust the experts.

• • •

Kathy Charmaz is a professor of sociology, has been touched by chronic illness in her family, and worked as an occupational therapist for a time. She saw firsthand the havoc that serious illness can cause in the lives of individuals and families. She believes the problem stems in part from our medical system itself. She wrote:

> *The combination of payment plans, patient-practitioner relationships, cultural beliefs, and medical ideologies produces an unwieldy and inflexible framework for thinking, acting, and feeling about illness. Practitioners usually treat those with chronic illnesses within a framework of care designed for those with acute illnesses, however inappropriate that framework is. Treating chronic illness within the acute care framework results in fragmented care, incomplete information, overburdened caregivers and isolated individuals left to handle the spiraling problems caused by illness as best they can.*[115]

We experienced what Dr. Charmaz describes in both direct and subtle ways: insurance companies that limited therapy as if I had an acute injury to recover from, not a chronic condition; medical institutions that rarely inquired about my psychological needs and didn't advocate for such care as an ordinary part of stroke recovery; little or no connection between groundbreaking research in the treatment of stroke during its immediate acute phase and research being done to improve rehabilitation for people well into the chronic stage of life after stroke.

Jim Indelicato had a particularly complicated medical situation after his stroke, and one of his daughters or wife was at his side nearly 24/7 in the weeks after. They closely watched everything about his care, listening to his doctors and asking them about anything that didn't seem to make sense. "Sometimes the nurses forget something," Diane remembered. "I would tell them, do not put that medicine in the wrong tube. They would go ahead and do it, and then he'd throw up and aspirate." She always tried to be friendly and respectful when intervening, but she never stopped participating.

"In Jim's medical report, we found out that the doctor wrote . . . 'listen to the family, they know what they're talking about,'" Diane shared with a smile. She really didn't get much push back to her constant questions and observations; over time, the staff accepted that she could be helpful. "We were there so much," she explained matter-of-factly. "We just know Jim."

Jim's daughter Joy, a professional counselor, made a mission of advocating for her father and researching his requirements and the latest breakthroughs in treatment. She asked his doctor about a recently developed full facial mask ventilator that might help her dad transition off the tracheostomy tube inserted directly into his neck through which he was breathing. With the trach he had at the time, he couldn't speak at all. Skeptical, the doctor said, "Joy, it won't work, but if you want to try it, you know what to look for." Since low oxygen levels can quickly cause confusion, Jim's family would be able to tell whether or not the new ventilator was working based on his behavior. It worked, and so did several other steps they tried that eventually led him to kick the ventilator completely four-and-a- half years after his stroke. Without such persistence on the part of his family, Jim is certain he wouldn't be where he is today.

Jim was fifty-nine when he had his stroke in 2010. He was ex-military and a thirty-two-time marathon finisher. He was fit, and his family knew he would fight for every bit of recovery he could possibly achieve. But lying on a bed with a ventilator and all kinds of tubes supporting him, it often felt to Diane as if nobody was looking past his immediate survival. "Jody said, 'Momma, bring a picture of how Daddy was, so they can see,'" Diane told me. She thought that conveying his former vitality might change how he was seen and treated. "I brought in a picture from his military service, in his blues, and one of him running a marathon," she continued. That was the beginning of their commitment to reminding everyone who was treating Jim that he would settle for nothing less than the most complete recovery possible. And it unquestionably helped, they say.

. . .

At my second stay at Stanford Hospital, I had the surgery to implant a stent in the cerebral portion of my carotid artery—the scariest part of my ordeal for my family. Not long later, Steve received a different kind of scare in the form of a letter from Blue Cross, our medical insurance provider at the time. Coverage for that entire stay at Stanford was denied because a stent implantation in a cerebral artery was experimental and so not covered, they said. The total in the column for "Patient Responsibility" was $990,000. Even though he knew it was ridiculous and that somehow we would get that decision reversed, the possibility of that kind of liability took his breath away.

Our experience and that of so many others drives home the fact that insurers often don't view the world through a lens of patient need but one that focuses on minimizing expenses. Anyone who doesn't fight hard to get the coverage they really want will invariably get less care than they should have, especially when it comes to rehabilitation services. We'd had the hassle of fixing insurance mistakes before, but then it didn't carry the same emotional burden of having to constantly fight with the system when we were already drowning in the overwhelming stress that a health emergency like stroke creates. At times, Steve felt as if the hospitals and Blue Cross were conspiring to make the system as complicated as possible. There were mistakes in billing or submissions to insurance. Hospitals filed for coverage long after the actual service. Insurers claimed that we used ancillary services that were out of network after we had specifically chosen the providers to keep everything in network. The list was endless. Steve wanted to spend his time supporting me and our kids, not sorting through, reconciling, and fighting medical paperwork.

Jodi Kravitz had been a good friend of Steve's since college, and she was part of his emotional support network. She asked him a simple but game-changing question: "Is there anyone else who could take that off your plate?" He decided to get help from a woman who supports people with health-care financial management as a business, and at a cost we could afford. Others I've spoken with have had an adult child or a very close friend who could take this extraordinarily time-consuming hassle off the primary caregiver's plate. The financial stakes are huge, and this support let Steve focus more of his time and attention where it was most needed—on me and our kids—without feeling irresponsible about the financial side of things.

$$\cdots$$

Cam Compton was in a tough financial situation about five years after her stroke. The insurance company that provided her long-term disability benefits just stopped making payments. They told her she no longer had a disability and could go back to work full time. She was working part time, but ongoing cognitive and physical challenges made longer days impossible. She knew she couldn't work full time because she had tried. Her doctors agreed. After months of fighting, she realized somewhat ironically that her cognitive disability was blocking her efforts to prove she actually had an ongoing disability. She hired a lawyer, and after nine months of no payments, the insurance company finally agreed to reinstate her coverage and pay her retroactively for the nine-month gap. The lawyer did help her win the battle, but at a significant cost: 20 percent of what she recovered.

Cam's story got even more interesting after that. She didn't realize that the agreement she had signed with the lawyer entitled him to 20 percent of all subsequent disability payments for three years. She's not clear about whether her cognitive disability caused her to miss that provision in the agreement, or her faulty memory led her to forget that she in fact understood and accepted it. But she couldn't deny that it was in the document she had signed. Six months after the successful reinstatement, she took a shot at regaining the lost income, and a few emails and phone calls with the attorney did the trick. He agreed he had been fairly compensated for his work and stopped taking anything out of her disability checks. "A great lesson," she explained. "You don't get what you don't ask for, and there are a lot of fair and caring people all around us."

Probably the most consistent frustration among stroke survivors is about the limits on insurance coverage for therapy. Mark Wells, a fifty-three-year-old African-American accountant in St. Louis when he had a stroke in 2013, had an incredibly frustrating experience with insurance. Covered by Medicaid at the time of his stroke, his benefits for therapy ran out very quickly. He was told that because of his disability he would gain coverage under Medicare. He explained, "But then I was told I had to be on disability for two years before that coverage would start. I think that's horrible . . . I've got a brain injury—it's not a cut on your arm or a broken leg. This is a brain injury, and they make us wait two years because we don't have the money to pay for therapy on our own. That's evil." Many survivors experience frustratingly limited care even with insurance, or they have to battle through strange coverage and requirements brought on by the bureaucracy of the medical system.

Manny Gigante said that although he's thankful for what he receives through Medicare, there's still a big gap in his coverage. "I don't qualify for MediCal," he said. "My wife's income and my disability payments put us over the cap. For seniors or someone over sixty-five, AARP can cover that gap, but for someone my age—forty-three this year—there isn't an answer." Manny is also a diabetic, which adds additional cost and complexity to getting the treatment he needs for recovery. Even if he did qualify for MediCal, California's Medicaid program for low-income people, he would have out-of-pocket costs over $600 per month, even for the reduced services he would get. Manny simply is not able to afford therapy that he knows would significantly improve his quality of life.

He also notes that some medical devices that are highly useful for survivors are no longer covered by insurers. "I actually use a SaeboFlex. When I first got evaluated for it back in 2003, insurance paid for it. My only out-of-pocket expense was like $30. Now, if a patient in 2016 wants to get that same device, they have to pay $1,200 out of pocket." As a result of the mounting costs and financial constraints, Manny stopped doing occupational and physical therapy for over ten years, only restarting recently. He tried to do some of it on his own with home programs, but he knows how much more he improves when he works with professionals.

When Kathy Howard lost the policy she had at work, she found one on the health-care marketplace that cost her $300 monthly with a $2,500 deductible. Not all the therapy she wanted was covered, but it wasn't bad. Then she received a notice that her monthly premium would be jumping up to $487. She decided to go shopping again and found a policy that was just $10 more per month, but her deductible more than doubled. "My therapy days are pretty much over until I get on Medicare," she told me. Unfortunately, we know from others that coverage for long-term stroke therapy under Medicare is not great. Like Manny, she was largely forced to take her therapy into her own hands. The table in her living room is filled with what she calls her self-therapy toolkit. It's frustrating because she, too, knows her progress would be better with professional help.

Sometimes, self-advocacy can lead to meaningful changes in coverage. Anthony Santos had some success when he found a therapist who was particularly helpful, but his insurance company declined coverage. After relentless pressure, he finally got them to cover the therapy—for a while. "They told me, 'Your brain's already healed; it's past a year and a half; there's nothing we can do for you,'" he quotes from a conversation with his insurance company. But at the same time, his therapist helped Anthony regain the ability to walk, then move his shoulder freely, then squat, bend, and more. "It's been more than three years since his stroke, and he's still regaining abilities," the therapist explained. Anthony couldn't afford to pay out of pocket for this therapy that was really changing his life. He kept battling and was able to extend coverage.

Initially, I had an insurance policy that had no absolute limit on the number of therapy sessions I could receive each year (an unusually good policy, I learned later) as long as they were medically necessary. Several times, the insurer claimed that the documentation of my continued progress did not meet the standard for "medically necessary." Each time that happened, many phone calls, documentation from my care team, and a formal appeal finally changed the ruling. But it took a ridiculous amount of time and energy.

As frustrating, incomplete, or insufficient as they might find it, every stroke survivor in this book has had medical insurance at the time of their stroke. That is not true for all people in the country. A Gallup-Healthways poll conducted in April 2017 found that 11.3 percent of U.S. adults didn't have health insurance in the first quarter of 2017, up about 4 percent from the third and fourth quarters of 2016.

• • •

This is an area where structural change is absolutely necessary, but it will require collective advocacy to change a system that will fight hard against the change. Insurance, especially around therapy, is set up as if our recovery is from a discrete injury rather than a long-term condition. Nearly every insurance policy limits therapy coverage to two or three times a week, for an hour each. Yet I've worked with many therapists and doctors who believe strongly that recovery from stroke would almost always be far faster and more complete if therapy was more intensive than that. Many policies have an annual cap of thirty covered sessions (four months at twice per week) for each kind of therapy, as if there is a standard recovery time and progression. Treating strokes like a typical injury, rather than the lifelong effort it is for many of us, is hindering how much recovery many survivors can make.

The practice of medicine in the United States is not organized to provide care. Incentives for hospitals, insurers, doctors, patients, drug companies, technology builders, companies, the government, taxpayers, and every other stakeholder are poorly aligned and out of date. Diane Indelicato was particularly frustrated with her experience of the health-care industry as one that seems to assume that a survivor just won't recover very much. Some of that relates to the data on improvement that is old and based on a time when most survivors were relatively old.

Luckily, there are people in our country working hard in politics, advocacy, and the medical system itself to understand and improve it. Several people in this book are working toward that goal. Through her book *Don't Leave Me This Way* and her speaking and advocacy work, Julia Fox Garrison is trying to do her part to improve health care. "As I was being churned through the system, I realized two things: I've got to show people that they can overcome the tragedy even in the face of being told they're going to die, and I've got to show the medical industry there's a *human being* inside of every patient, because sometimes the bureaucracy and all the policies and procedures overshadow the actual person." She points out that just two decades ago, there was really no concept of patient-centered care, and although the medical industry is beginning to shift in that direction, we have a long way to go. "It still is clouded by bureaucracy, and policy, and procedure, and code," Julia said. "And that's the problem."[116]

The days, months, and early years after a stroke are often the hardest and most stressful for a survivor and his or her family. Their lives are made even more difficult by having to navigate complicated foreign terrain like hospitals, therapy programs, and insurance providers. It can be easy to assume that in this time of need, health-care professionals will make sure survivors get the best care available. Despite the good intentions of so many individuals, our medical system makes that the exception, not the rule. As survivors, we, and our families and other supporters, have to take ownership for our own care, engage constructively with care professionals, and, when necessary, fight for the best we can get.

ADVOCATING IN THE U.S. MEDICAL SYSTEM:
CHAPTER 16 HIGHLIGHTS

- Survivors have to be their own advocate in our system—both to get the best possible care and the most possible support from insurance.

- The American medical system is not organized to deliver optimal care and compassion to patients.

- Medical professionals are usually well intentioned and capable, but they are often overworked; nobody cares about your care as much as you and your family, friends, and supporters.

- Most care providers are very receptive to questions asked nicely and with respect—don't defer too much to "the professionals."

- Survivors must also advocate for more support through insurance, which unfortunately has incentives to stop payments and coverage; you can change their minds.

PART THREE:

REDEFINING
Recovery

CHAPTER 17.

Reclaiming the Basics

O n September 24, 2010, Danny had visited Valley Medical to watch
Jonathan, my new speech therapist, coax out my first poststroke words
with familiar songs and help me sing my own name. Steve found out about the
breakthrough later and recorded his experience of it on CaringBridge that night.

> *I got wind of this great progress when Danny called me, and he sent me*
> *a short iPhone video he took of the "My name is Debra Meyerson" bit.*
> *But my elation didn't fully hit until Marcia called me at about 2:30,*
> *put Deb on the phone, and with a little coaching I could hear in the*
> *background, I heard a very clear "I love you, Steve"!*
>
> *Quite a sight I must have been sitting in my office, weeping*
> *unabashedly as, with the pattern Danny described, she repeated*
> *that several times, increasingly quickly and with delight in her*
> *voice, until she faded with exhaustion.*

My stroke had sent me to the very bottom of Maslow's hierarchy of needs.
I could no longer take for granted the most basic aspects of life: a properly
functioning body, safety in everyday situations, the capacity to secure food
and shelter, and the ability to communicate my needs to others. Recovering
those functions was the sole focus for my family and me at the very beginning.
I remember that moment in Valley Medical so distinctly not only because I
had reclaimed some speech but also because I had regained another human
necessity: I could tell my husband how much I loved him.

For most stroke survivors, our early recovery is laser focused on rebuilding foundations. We need to learn anew how to walk, speak, and swallow. When our most basic needs are not fulfilled, very little else matters. These are the foundation of Maslow's pyramid, on which everything else rests. Yet, single-minded focus on the basics cannot lead to a meaningful life. We also need to build a life beyond those survival basics, to fulfill other needs.

For many of us, we will battle physical disabilities for the rest of our lives. This is true regardless of how much progress we make and how much effort we put into our recovery. After the initial battle for survival and stability, we need to redefine recovery more broadly than overcoming specific deficiencies. Recovery isn't about getting back to exactly who we were. Instead, the goal is to reclaim the pieces that mean the most to us.

This forces us to examine what matters most in that recovery. For many of us, that means building more self-confidence and independence, and finding a level of stability in the most basic requirements of life. That creates the foundation on which we can focus on higher needs and the process of rebuilding a rewarding life. In *Being Mortal: Illness, Medicine and What Matters in the End*, Atul Gawande notes, "Our most cruel failure in how we treat the sick and the aged is the failure to recognize that they have priorities beyond merely being safe and living longer; the chance to shape one's story is essential to sustaining meaning in life."[117] Rather than point ourselves blindly at everything in our old life, we can focus on the efforts that will be most helpful in building a rewarding life going forward.

· · ·

After my stroke, I felt broken. So did Sean Maloncy, who articulated the jarring recognition that everything can fail. So did Anthony Santos, who wondered when stroke might strike again, and Jim Indelicato, who found himself fearful for himself and his family when he couldn't be the fixer and protector. So, too, for Ahaana Singh, who felt she couldn't keep up mentally and others just didn't understand. Professor Sharon Kaufman observed, "In the year following the stroke, no person we spoke with, even those who had visibly and tangibly regained lost function, claimed to have recovered."[118] How much of us is lost, we wonder, and will we get it back? And will we break again?

It's hard to make sense of such a sudden loss of function. A gulf emerges between the pre-stroke body and the poststroke body. "An individual enters a completely new world, experiencing fundamental physiological as well as physical challenges," observed the authors of poststroke narratives. "The body becomes something foreign and separate from the self. The discovery that no cure is available comes as a shock."[119] This is one of the distinguishing features of stroke: the symptoms can be treated, but there is no cure available or recovery guaranteed. It's hard to process this new reality.

This experience is made even more difficult by the uncertainty of rehab. "The process of rehab is unknown to the patient," said occupational therapist Waleed Al-Oboudi. "It's not clear to clinicians either. The patient is actually beginning a process that is very, very difficult to define and navigate. We could ask ten clinicians and get ten different answers." After most injuries, traumas, or surgeries there is a relatively well-defined recovery expectation. This is not true at all for strokes. The closest thing to a standard in the medical community is the extremely unfortunate mantra that most recovery happens in the first twelve months. Thankfully, that myth is losing credibility.

The lack of clarity about the future is stressful. It becomes hard to balance acceptance of the situation with determination to push rehab hard, both of which are important. "I want to give myself a break from pushing forward, but it's easier said than done. You put a lot more pressure on yourself than anybody else does," said Ahaana Singh. After stroke, the brain is already traumatized, so more anxiety can actually hurt the recovery. "The brain is affected in the patient's level of tenseness. If a patient is, and rightly so, feeling down in a situational depression, that affects their recruitment to and participation in the therapy." said Waleed Al-Oboudi.

In the face of the uncertainty about recovery, survivors can become overwhelmed by the amount to be done. But focusing on small wins and just the next step can support both mental health and physical rehab. We must remaster basics before we can try things that are more complex. In education, this is referred to as scaffolding. When I told Steve I loved him from Valley, I needed cues from my mother to speak the words. In hindsight, I realize I was not actually speaking as we typically think of it. I was recreating the physical ability to form words, not really working the speech center of my brain. But mimicking was the first level of the scaffold—I couldn't speak original thoughts until I could manipulate my lips and tongue and voice to control sound.

It was probably a good thing I didn't realize at the time that my "I love you" wasn't genuine speech. My trainers knew that celebrating an early success—mimicking a sentence—was both necessary and motivating. Focusing on one step at a time let me build speech back up in a more productive way than if I'd attempted spontaneous speech immediately. "Once a small win has been accomplished, forces are set in motion that favor another small win. When a solution is put in place, the next solvable problem becomes more visible," wrote Karl Weick.[120]

As we push ahead with determination and focus, progress and motivation build on each other. Anthony Santos's mother Martina, who helped her son recover from his stroke, observed, "Now that he's starting to see the results, he's not sad anymore; he doesn't get as frustrated anymore. Even though he would like it to be quicker!" It is crushingly frustrating when we look at where we are and compare ourselves with who we were when we were at the peak of our previous functionality. "You have to keep hope," said Anthony. "Once you lose hope, that would really be the end of life."

Randy Miller's wife Rose shares the same forward-thinking attitude when it comes to her husband's stroke recovery. It didn't happen immediately, though, and it was thanks to a supportive physician that they became aware that there could be a long road to recovery. "At our very first stroke support meeting, we met Dr. Hubbard. We looked like the deer in the headlights. After introducing himself, the very first thing he said was not to believe the doctors about the six months or one year to recover. He said that people improve years after their stroke. We felt a burden lifted off our shoulders at that moment. It still gives us hope about continuing to recover." Rose said that being with Randy over the three years after his stroke was like "Watching pieces fall into place. There were blank spaces, then all of a sudden, a piece would drop in."

If what we truly care about is regaining our basic functions, independence, and lives, then we can't focus on how far we've fallen. Instead, we look up and climb one rung of the ladder at a time. As Jim Indelicato told survivors at his rehab center, "Why did you have a stroke? Who cares? That's history. Now you just make it better for tomorrow."

• • •

As we struggle with rehab, we are also challenged with questions about how our physical deficits redefine us. As people, we do not separate our body from our selves. "The notion of mind/body separation, though a strong epistemological tradition in American culture, is not a lived reality for the patient," writes Professor Kaufman. While we may talk of a soul, spiritual self, or mind, our experience is that the brain and body and self are inextricably linked. "The impaired and restricted body . . . significantly threatens the conception of an intact and autonomous self." It is hard to overcome the feeling of having a broken body that is no longer trusted to do the bidding of the mind.

Having to rely on others makes you question everything. Julia Fox Garrison felt this acutely. "Initially, the most important thing that I lost was my independence. And we're talking right down to the basics, not talking about independent like you want to go to a movie independently. I'm talking about having someone feed me. Having two people put me on a toilet, having someone wipe my ass. Those are things that make you go through this period of thinking, 'What am I? Am I just an object?'"

Kaufman sums up the feelings well:

> *For patients and families I observed, "failure," "vulnerability," "anger," and "humiliation" characterize that experience. What threatens them is not the disease alone, as it is medically defined and treated, but rather the existential awareness of loss, distortion, fear, and entrapment that emerges sometimes long after the patient's condition is medically stable.*[121]

In Kaufman's study, one participant said, "You can't imagine how frustrating it is when you are dependent on all these people for your every move. It's like you're not a person. What if they decide not to come?"[122] The degree and nature of independence becomes a defining part of recovering both basic functions and a sense of self. Very few people seek truly complete independence—we want to be interdependent with our family, friends, and colleagues for a healthy and social life. But nobody wants to need help to eat and poop. Finding the appropriate balance can be challenging to both the survivor and their supporters.

I often found that people around me were unsure of how and how much to help me. Do they jump up to help me set the table, seeing how much more difficult it is for me, or will that incur the wrath of the fiercely, stubbornly independent Deb? Understanding the journey we are going through can help others walk it with us, rather than guess in the dark. I watched this dialogue take form several times in talking to other survivors and their families. "I can't relax knowing you're over there struggling," said Julia's husband Jim. She responded, "Don't you understand? I want to be independent. I want to do this. I need to accomplish this."

They recalled this exchange later with a deeper understanding that her goals as a stroke survivor change what's important about the situation. "He's thinking 'most women would love this,' and I'm insisting, 'I know, but most women aren't in the situation of trying to improve their independence.'" It is not about grasping onto independence for its own sake, trying to pretend we can do everything the way we used to. As part of our recovery, we need to keep building small steps toward independent function—these small, seemingly insignificant victories help us continue moving forward and focus on the next achievable goal. The small steps add up.

We need support in this process, and often that means letting us struggle. Danny's friend Kayla Cornale works with athletes with disabilities for the Canadian Paralympic team. She has a simple guideline for how she supports them. She may be the one person in their lives who won't move a muscle to offer help until they ask for it. "Does that mean every once in a while, someone will struggle and get frustrated, and maybe think I'm being thoughtless? Sure. I can live with that," she said. "For every one of those, there are a few dozen more who feel emotional support—that I believe they don't need help, that they can do it themselves, and that they get to test their limits." Stroke survivors are in a similar place. Often those around us see that we've fallen off the ladder and, meaning well, want to carry us back to the top. But it's more important for us to rebuild our ability to climb the ladder ourselves, even if we can't get all the way to the top.

Of course, at times we will need more support getting up even the first steps of the ladder. Whether immediately after stroke or in the longer term for those with significant disabilities, many of us must come to grips with more dependence on others than we are comfortable with. Many survivors feel guilty at the weight they impose on others. Even in my earliest recovery days, I felt shame that I was pulling my children away from school. Dr. Venkat has seen many parents or spouses in particular who struggle with similar shame. "It's almost like a complete 360-degree turn. I'm not the provider now, and that's bad enough," Jim Indelicato shared. "But in addition, I'm a burden on someone else. That comes with a huge sense of shame. It's like we both had a stroke," he said of his wife. She disagreed. She is happy to take on more so he can focus on recovery, and takes huge pride in how far he's come.

In all the interviews I did—and most were very frank—I found that stroke survivors worried about the negative impact and burden on others far more than their families did. Of course, there are exceptions. There are moments when supportive families explode in frustration, and there are spouses—like Mary Jones's—who just give up. But based on my experience and that of my interviewees, most families embrace the role of supporter.

Psychologist Melanie Drane's sister had a massive stroke. She describes, "the strange gift of hard times. In spite of the hardship, some relationships become much more intimate." That doesn't make it easy, and at first, every survivor feels like a burden. "It's an enormous challenge to figure out how to make sense of things once they've been thrown into chaos by a stroke," she writes. But through the process of learning, redesigning relationships, and recovering together, this can change. Laure Wang, the survivor with locked-in syndrome, wrote in her book *Reflections on a Changed Life*, "Because of my stroke, [my husband] could now experience firsthand the hardest job you could ever love [taking care of the kids]."

Our supporters, like the survivors themselves, have good reason to be bitter or resentful at times, as their lives have also become more difficult. But they, too, can bounce forward. Under some circumstances, stroke support groups provide a community in which the discourse facilitates renegotiation of identity for both persons with aphasia and their significant others.

So as guilty as we may feel for "burdening" others, making use of our support system can deepen our relationships. Along with all the challenges, stroke can become a growth experience for all involved. Communities, friendships, and relationships grow significantly stronger from overcoming adversity together.

• • •

Early in my recovery, I was determined that my stroke would take nothing from me. When I first began replying to email, I had Steve help me craft replies that sounded fluent, but I stopped him from mentioning that he had helped me write them or indicate that my stroke had hindered me much at all. I wanted to pretend that in the longer scheme of things, it wouldn't be a factor. Over time, I relaxed. I now make it clear I am getting help, or I write simple replies myself. I don't put in my contact lenses as much anymore because it's easier to wear glasses. I frequently choose my exercise for the day based on what is easiest to make happen, not what I'd most prefer. These may seem like small, obvious steps. But for me, it was a leap to reassess the reality of my situation and make choices based on that reality. I'm not doing something different than what I really want to do; I'm deciding what I want to do based on my life today, not my life before the stroke.

In the aftermath of stroke, we are forced to reassess what is most important to us in our new situation, and to prioritize and adapt. Kathy Howard wears a bracelet that says, "Thriving is Surviving." She doesn't want to just chase her missing capabilities. She wants to thrive as a person, to spend her time on the things that matter and make her feel she is thriving. So her recovery is focused not on blindly recovering function but on enabling the things that matter. She said, "I'm a stroke survivor. I need to stand up and say, 'You know what? It's going to be different.' That's something we don't necessarily want to hear—that life will be different." Our lives and selves are always changing, and with trauma like stroke, we are forced to change far more quickly. That is daunting, but luckily, we are remarkably adaptable given the right approach.

During a writing session for this book in 2018, my son Danny was home when I came back from getting some exercise. "Did you just go for a walk?" he asked. "No, swim," I said. He asked who I went with, knowing that in the last few years, trips to the pool included nearby friends like Kim Menninger or Karen Jordan. After a few tries, I successfully told him I went by myself. He was surprised—a few years ago, I had desperately wanted to swim solo but had accepted the fact that I needed support to get ready and get safely into the pool. I had started swimming solo about eight months before, seven years after I first got in the water shortly after my stroke.

My notion of independence had changed. I am, in fact, able to handle most aspects of a pool trip on my own. But I still can't put on a swim cap and goggles by myself. Earlier, that stopped me from going alone. But my speech is better, and I've gotten to know enough of the workers at the local pool that I can get the last bit of help once I'm there. And while my greater abilities are part of it, even more important is that I've gotten comfortable asking even people I don't know for help. For me, swimming is a good example of the journey. First, I could swim with Steve's help and his intimate knowledge of my needs. Then, I went with a close friend, who could work with me through the frustration and issues. With a little more time, I could do it with other friends, and eventually with the help of any worker on duty or a fellow swimmer at the pool. Small win by small win, I regained my independence, albeit slightly redefined. But, after all, none of us is ever truly independent, as we all need others in our lives.

When people ask my family how I'm doing and if I'm recovered, they say we are living happily in our "new normal." Is my life harder than it was? Yes. Are theirs? Also, yes. Do I rely on them for things we all wish I could do myself? Yes. But with hard work, many small wins, and lots of support, I have regained much function and independence. I can walk. I can do pretty much anything that can be done with one hand, including drive. I can't tie my shoes by myself, but I found elastic lace replacements that allow me to slip them on one-handed.

Have I recovered? I've regained nowhere near my full, pre-stroke capabilities. But I no longer fear that my basic needs won't be met and rarely need help to meet them. I have recovered in a way that I can focus more of my efforts, and my requests for support, further up Maslow's pyramid: building a sense of belonging, purpose, and fulfillment in my new life. I now think of my recovery more in the context of these goals, not just regaining my capabilities.

CHAPTER 18.

Choice in Our New Identities

British writer Robert McCrum was struck down by a stroke at age forty-two and wrote about the aftermath. "The cruel fact is that this former self is irretrievably shattered into a thousand pieces, and try as one may to glue those pieces back together again, the reconstituted version will never be better than a cracked, imperfect assembly, a constant mockery of one's former, successful individuality."[123] I understand McCrum. His words vividly capture how I feel at times. But only at times, only on my bad days.

How we move forward after stroke is a choice. Comparing ourselves to our former, successful individuality is only one of many lenses we can look through, and it's probably not the best. Stroke can limit our options, but it does not seal our fate. It is our choice: do we reject our stroke and fight like hell to recover our old life, accept it passively, or embrace the stroke as part of our life and carve a new path with that reality as part of our landscape?

For our entire lives, we have been building narratives about who we are. This continuous story is the core of our identity. It makes us "us," even as we grow and change, sometimes dramatically. "Identities are formed through efforts to develop a coherent, continuous biography, where a person's life story is the sensible result of a series of related events or cohesive themes," wrote Sally Maitlis in "Who Am I Now?"[124] But a trauma like stroke interrupts that story, jarringly. Stroke knocks us off the path we had been on our entire lives. Our new situation wasn't even in the set of possibilities we thought existed for our life before.

We've built relationships, affiliations, activities, and personalities—a lifetime of experiences and memories that, consciously and subconsciously, tell us who we are. Stroke throws a wrench in that: relationships are changed; activities, jobs, and careers may be lost; goals and plans are pushed out of reach. "Medical sociologists have suggested that when people acquire a chronic illness certain life stories are interrupted, the sense of coherence is undermined, and the future becomes uncertain and unpredictable," write Caroline Ellis-Hill and Sandra Horn from the University of Southampton.[125] This threatens the survivor's sense of belonging, self-esteem, and feelings of control over their own life and future. The psychological needs Maslow describes in the middle sections of the pyramid are disrupted.

From this trauma comes confusion and resentment, but also opportunity. In the Japanese art of *kintsugi*, broken pottery is repaired with gold or silver, mending the cracks. This creates a new piece that doesn't hide the cracks, instead celebrating trauma as an important part of the piece's history. Survivors are presented with the chance to be thoughtful about how we want to rebuild our lives and make something fulfilling as we mend ourselves. As the proverb suggests, "Necessity is the mother of invention." Forced by stroke to reinvent ourselves, we can do so with a lifetime's worth of experience and perspective about who we want to be for the rest of our lives. I like to think I had more wisdom at fifty-three when faced with the need to rebuild my adult life than I did at eighteen, when I started doing so for the first time.

"Pressure builds diamonds," says another relevant proverb. We may have fewer options after a stroke, and may face greater adversity, but that gives us the chance to channel our energy into the few things we truly care most about. We have the opportunity to reevaluate what matters and why, and we have the ability to decide who we will become. Our lives evolve over time anyway. Following a stroke, we are forced into more dramatic change, so we might as well take the opportunity to shape its direction.

• • •

"Many people are surprised that I celebrate my stroke anniversary," said Julia Fox Garrison. "But for me, it is cause for celebration because I'm still here. It allows me to thump my chest and say I won. I've enjoyed twenty more years of being a wife, mother, daughter, sister, and friend, and I'm still going strong." Julia still suffers from a limp and disabilities on her left side, but she unequivocally declares, "I won." To her, beating stroke is not about recovering all her function but about coming through the adversity to spend her life on the things she cares most about: being a wife, mother, daughter, sister, friend, and now passionate health-care advocate.

It is a cliché that those who suffer a tragedy or trauma are reminded of what really matters in life. But there is a lot of truth in clichés. Events like the death of a loved one often stimulate reflection and reevaluation. Too often, these lessons fade as people return to their day-to-day routines. For stroke survivors, though, we often do not have the luxury of returning to our day-to-day routines. We continue to improve, but reckoning with our disabilities on a daily basis forces us to continually reflect and reevaluate. Everything we do might be harder, our time and energy scarcer and more precious. So we are forced to choose what we care most about and put effort into as we create our new story. Maitlis says, "Of particular importance in this process is the story or narrative, which provides the central means through which people construct, describe, and understand their experiences, and through this, their identities."[126] We can choose to use our disrupted life as an opportunity to deliberately ask ourselves what we really care most about, what we want to do in the future, and what that means for our story going forward.

That was true for many of the survivors whose stories contribute to this book. Mark Wells observed, "You're so busy grinding. Working all the time. I gotta go to work, to pay the bills, to do this, to do that, get some food on the table . . . When you fall off that treadmill and start looking around, it kind of shakes you all up. You take stock and say, 'What's really going on here?' You get a whole different perspective on life." Mark built a new identity for himself after his stroke by exploring his cultural roots, contemplating his spirituality, and for the first time being unafraid to challenge many things he had been told all his life and simply accepted as true. His stroke launched him on a deep and incredibly rewarding personal exploration.

The benefits of embracing the opportunity to make significant life changes after trauma are often more clear to those who have been through challenging circumstances before. José Cofiño was a good friend of Steve's in graduate school. He had been battling ALS for five years when we last spoke, and he passed away two months later. As his disease became more severe, José and his partner had to work through how to make sense of his deteriorating condition, make use of the time they had left, and enjoy life as much as they could in the unchangeable situation.

José had struggled with identity issues before. He felt anguish during the many years he had concealed that he was gay. He worried about how family, colleagues, friends, and classmates would respond. When he finally came out several years after finishing graduate school, the complete acceptance he experienced was a turning point. He said at that point he learned to fully embrace his identity.

When he was diagnosed with ALS about twenty years later, he and his partner made a very conscious decision to be open and public about their journey, hoping their story would help others with the disease. After about a year of "being in shock," they decided they wanted to retain control and make clear choices about how to spend their remaining time. They knew that ALS would eventually take José's life, but it hadn't yet. They founded Beyond ALS and dedicated themselves to increasing awareness for ALS and raising funds to help find a solution. José pushed past the many instincts to recede from social life and let his disease shape him. Instead, he seized control and shared what he was learning with others. He shared his story at his reunion shortly after his ALS diagnosis. José told us that the class became one of his most crucial support networks as he made sense of that final journey. The unanticipated benefit of his decision was that his class bonded in new ways in their efforts to support him. In asking for support, he also gave a great gift to people he cared about.

. . .

"You are the average of your five closest friends," said Jim Rohn, the author and entrepreneur who mentored famous self-help guru Tony Robbins. The science behind this claim may be a bit vague, but few of us dispute the impact that those closest to us have on experience and happiness in life. They are probably a pretty good reflection of who we are. Healthy relationships are the single most important factor in long-term happiness. Choosing who we spend time with—whether at each day's lunch or in lifelong partnerships—is the most important set of choices we make in our lives.[127]

Inevitably, relationships change after stroke. A few people will disappoint; a few will astound. Some friendships will tighten, and others will drift. Most will simply evolve. But as these changes are taking place, we can each ask ourselves: what do I want out of my relationships? Who do I most want to surround me? Why?

I had to grow into this realization. A few years ago, I felt more pain about my faded relationships with former colleagues, like those who ran the Center on Philanthropy and Civil Society with me. We had been close, shared interests, and supported each other for years. Yet in my new life, very removed from theirs, we had less reason to be close. We drifted apart. This is no indictment of them or of me. Time is limited, and friendships take work—not all of them can be first priority. They still matter to me, and I think I still matter to them as well. I have simply grown more comfortable with the idea that our being less close isn't bad; it's just a reflection of our new reality.

I now value relationships with my closest friends more than ever. Often, these friendships go back decades, with many shared experiences to build on, which helps us communicate effectively and deeply despite my aphasia. This deep connection is now harder in big group settings, so I've shrunk my circles and social events a bit. That's how I've chosen to adapt my social world, given my own preferences and needs for belonging and close relationships. Says identity expert Barbara Shadden, "Because identities are constituted in social interaction, they must be negotiated in a social context to be accepted as legitimate."[128] Through my changing relationships and affiliations, I've rediscovered and reconstructed who I am post stroke.

Laure Wang's choices have been completely different, because her identity and goals are different. She has always had an active social life and a wide, vibrant group of friends. She draws energy from these social bonds and loves the camaraderie of a big group. She doesn't want to give that up, and although speech is much harder for her than it is for me, it means a lot for her to simply be in the room. So rather than change her social circles, she's changed how she interacts with them and what role she brings to the group: "Before I would have been talking and not listening. Now, I listen."

Since her stroke, Julia Fox Garrison has also refocused herself on her relationships. "I think I'm a kinder person. I was a nice person before, but I think I'm a kinder person having gone through what I've been through and needing to have kindness toward me. Kindness is so underrated, and it's so free and easy to give. I think I've become a better person." She actively works to be a better friend, play her role in her family, and help other stroke survivors.

Like the individuals we choose to spend time with, the communities we choose to be a part of can both reflect and influence the person we want to become. In *The Art of Community,* Charles Vogl describes member identity as the shared values and motivations that bond members in a community.[129] By participating in a community, members understand their own identity better. Our communities and affiliations are as varied as we are, and so are our reactions to them and theirs to us after stroke.

Some survivors turn deeper into their religious groups, or neighborhoods, or their extended families. Some pick up new hobbies, and a large number are inspired to volunteer more of their time, often to help other stroke survivors. Participating in community activities, even just meetings, is often harder than before, so survivors are often more selective in what they do and become very committed to their causes. Dr. Venkat points out, "People find a different meaning in their life. I don't see that very early on after stroke. It happens toward the second year . . . People give back more to the community, volunteer, start survivor groups, write books." They are learning to live their values in their new circumstance, and to play an active role shaping their evolving identity.

Many in this book have embraced the stroke survivor community, and yet even that varies widely based on what each person is looking for. Sean Maloney sought a cause where he could have an impact on stroke prevention, trying to develop technology that would help identify arterial blockages early on. Randy and Rose sought companionship and founded a stroke survivor Meetup group that is now very active. Jim sought to motivate others who'd experienced trauma, and he leads them by example at Paraquad. Kathy sought a community to help, and she assists other survivors one-on-one and by organizing events. I sought a new way to share knowledge to benefit others, a lifelong passion of mine, and embraced the stroke survivor community as one that I might help.

. . .

A few years after my stroke, I was no longer exclusively focused on recovery, and was trying to craft my new life. I wanted to orient my rehab around health and relationships. I had reflected on what I cared about and made some changes. I was still working hard on my rehab, but emotionally I was struggling. I was pushing the mythological boulder up the hill, and I wasn't even sure what hill I was on, how high it was, or why I needed to get to the top. My priorities felt abstract, not real, and not part of my daily life. I was still trying to reclaim everything, but I did not feel like I was reclaiming anything.

"Goal setting is part of being healthy mentally," my primary care physician Sarah Watson told me. I needed more tangible achievements that tied my day-to-day work to what I cared most about long term. "Having goals and having an ability to work really hard toward something are things that make people stronger and healthier and probably help them do things that no one ever thought they could do." I began to shape my rehab around specific goals I had in my life. Physical therapy was to prepare myself for walking and riding a horse in Peru. Speech therapy was to practice the presentation I'd be giving to pitch this book. Rosetta Stone sessions gave way to responding to emails on my own. Dr. Watson believes that having milestone goals helped me regain much more speech than anybody expected.

Julia Fox Garrison looks back on her own journey in a similar way. There was an initial period during which she just tried to get back as much as she could, and then another period where she got better every day if she just set her sights on accomplishing things she cared about. She's currently working on two personal goals: a memoir and a TEDTalk to spread her message about thinking in a positive manner.

Goals are an important part of development across domains and situations. They are particularly relevant to stroke survivors, who must balance the frustratingly long arc of recovery with the need for painfully slow, small wins. A commonly used framework cites three criteria for good working goals: that they be specific, realizable, and immediate (near-term).

These features give people clarity about what they should be working on, motivation that it can be achieved before burnout, and short feedback loops to learn and reenergize for future goals. "If people work for something concrete, if they have an opportunity for visible success from which they can draw confidence, and if people can translate their excitement and optimism into immediate action, then a small win is probable, as is their heightened interest in attempting a second win,"[130] wrote Karl Weick.

Sean Maloney went through a similar process. "I had to learn to speak again," he recalled. "It was so hard. So hard. I've got a video I recorded two months after my stroke. The video was me trying to say, 'Get the camera on me.' I couldn't say it. I couldn't say it." He said this looking backward, having improved his speech dramatically since then. His improvements came through determination, but also through strategically setting goals—not just for speech but for many parts of his life.

"He'll always be involved in something," said his therapist, Lisa, talking about the ambitious goals Sean sets. He now advocates for stroke survivors and uses that mission to guide his rehab. In his previous life, he was a "true orator," said Lisa, with "the gift of gab." In rebuilding himself, he's had to both reconstruct his ability to speak and change the way he approaches that part of his life. He used to do everything unscripted, in the moment, full of personality. But in his recovery from the stroke, that hasn't always been possible—a monologue that worked fine one day might get stuck the next. When he gives speeches now, he reluctantly uses a script. "I want you to be able to add your personality back into it," Lisa told him. "But you also need to have something in case you are not able to do that."

Given his personality and his goals, he does push himself to go it alone, but he now accepts a script as a backup. "I think putting yourself out there in situations where you might not succeed really does something," said Lisa. Sean is striving for something that he cares about, that defines him, but he does it one step at a time. Thinking back to the video of himself struggling to speak years ago, he said, "I think this video is perfect because it's me. I've looked at it lots of times subsequently, and thankfully, it's in the past. Tomorrow is better than today. Every day, tomorrow is better than today."

It's not easy to adopt Julia and Sean's positive attitudes, and it is nearly impossible in the period right after stroke, when everything feels like a deficit. Recent survivors seldom talked about gaining a higher sense of consciousness or greater understanding of the world, says Professor Kathy Charmaz. Nor did they share revelations about themselves or insights they gained into human nature from their recovery experiences. But as stroke survivors mature in their recovery, they begin to make choices about what they prioritize and how to pursue goals that reflect these priorities. That has a huge impact: personal goals; a positive, hopeful attitude; progress in rehab; and self-improvement all go hand in hand. Charmaz found "a striking contrast" between recent survivors working desperately to recover lost capabilities and "those who had improved and no longer suffered as greatly as they had in the past. These individuals were more likely to see their earlier suffering as a path to knowledge and self-discovery."[131]

• • •

This evolution comes with time, but it is something that I think survivors must choose to undertake. Our stroke happened; do we want to reject, accept, or embrace that fact? Like Malik, a few survivors I spoke to for this book are stuck in the first stage of the journey. They are looking back at the path they fell from and are not yet examining the path they want to build going forward. They struggle to maintain old relationships or lament the loss of them. They don't pursue new relationships because they see only the loss of what made their lives meaningful before the stroke. They don't feel the belonging or accomplishment that make life fulfilling.

They feel estranged from others and from themselves. Nearly all of us were in this stage for a period.

Mark Wells was initially depressed after his stroke, too. He remembers thinking that he didn't care if he died. But one day while watching a TV program about biblical stories, he switched his perspective. "You know what?" he thought. "I just got to learn how to be content. If this is my destiny, then I know my creator is going to give me everything that I need to survive this, but I just have to learn how to be content." He decided to accept his stroke and work within its limitations.

Most survivors I talked to had accepted, even embraced, their strokes. They are building new lives that follow the contours of the old, but with conscious adjustments. Most of their core values and the anchor traits in their personal narratives are similar to the old ones, but the ways they are exhibited have changed. "I am still a driven person; I am still a stubborn person," said Manny Gigante. "But I know that I have to take on a more creative role in my life . . . I can't go along in the same way I was before."

Jim Indelicato loved being the fixer, the coach, the family provider, and the leader that he had been with the U.S. Air Force. After his stroke, he struggled with the loss of these roles. The man who directed fitness for a military group now struggled with using his wheelchair by himself. He could no longer repair things around the house. But listening to his family speak, it's clear that Jim has found ways to live out the values he found so important in those earlier roles: persistence, discipline, family, and leadership by example. He walks his family through how to fix the things he used to fix, building their skills.

"It is so inspiring to watch him—it's like nothing I've ever seen," said his wife Diane. "He's by far the most determined person I've ever known." His kids chimed in that he's teaching his grandkids just by his determination and the example he sets. "He's still so valuable to the world, to the people he's influenced," they said. They talked about the therapist who invited him to her wedding, a kid at the hospital who complained and got motivation from Jim, and how he spends extra time at training facilities helping and inspiring others.

Diane always thought of him as her superman. He didn't want to lose that, so he turned his situation into an opportunity to put even more focus on the parts of his life that mattered most. "The influence is just beyond anything. He was an amazing person before the stroke and will be remembered for that, but the stroke is his legacy—what he has done through this terrible thing that happened that nobody knows why." Jim now spends more time with family and less with colleagues. He spends more time on rehab than on training. But Jim still derives belonging, love, and meaning from the same sources that always defined him. His commitment to his values brought the family closer together than ever. "It's one of the positives, many positives, in my mind," said his daughter Joy.

Some survivors recognize and embrace the opportunity to change more dramatically through the recovery process. It's so easy to follow a path through life without designing it yourself, and for some, the wake-up call is worth the painful interruption of life and even some lingering disabilities. Kathy Howard said, "I'm not the same person I was before. I'm kind of glad [the stroke] stole that person." Although most survivors aren't quite that positive about their experience—at least not all the time—it reflects the very real truth that the constraints of stroke recovery can force us to build a life that matters more and is more rewarding than the life we might have otherwise followed. Such a large dose of forced perspective can sometimes be a blessing. Charmaz found that for many chronically ill people, the illness became "a tool of self-discovery and a fundamental source of later self-development."[132]

I used to find belonging through close family, strong and supportive friendships, and professional groups dedicated to the same issues I care deeply about. All of those felt threatened after my stroke. But eight years in,

I appreciate how these bonds have held strong and evolved, even if I never would have chosen this path. I still regret that I couldn't be a more involved mother to my high school daughter, but my kids grew up faster and stronger because of my stroke. We are closer, as a family, than ever. It's harder for me to participate in some conversations and activities, so some of my friendships are more distant. Other friendships have evolved and allow me to feel comfortable just the way I am. More than ever, I know I am loved by my closest friends, and I know the importance of supporting and loving them. I've lost some sense of belonging in the academic circles I used to travel, and I've lost some friends from that world. That hurts. But as I take stock, I realize that the communities that matter most to me—the May Meaning Meeting, for example—still welcome me. And I've gained new communities, like those connected to boards on which I now serve—the Peninsula Stroke Association and Bay Area Women's Sports Initiative—that reflect my values and evolving goals.

I always prided myself on being independent, an athlete, a feminist, a sailor. All of these identities are now harder to live out in the way I'd like, of course. But the recovery journey has helped me see each in a new light. For a few years after my stroke, I chafed at my increased dependence. My daughter's Chapel Talk helped me realize that none of us are ever truly independent— humans can't work that way. We crave relationships, partnerships, support— we are in this together. The nature of my activities has changed, requiring more physical help than before. Accepting that as my new reality lets me focus on independence in a productive and (slightly) less stubborn way. I can't run, give academic talks at conferences, or sail small sailboats on my own. I miss all three. But once I gave up mourning those losses, I was able to build back my ability to get the underlying value of each: I can now swim or walk or bike to pump endorphins; I can push gender issues by supporting old colleagues and sharing their work; and I can coach my children to adjust the sails so we can still enjoy the relaxation of sailing as a family.

I also still consider myself a teacher. I want to create and share knowledge. This book has been my attempt to do that, regaining a part of my life after my career as a professor was taken away. Writing this book has been among the hardest things I've ever done. It put me face-to-face with my past experiences, at times making it hard to take my own advice about looking forward. I have been reliant on my early partner Sally, who did the lion's share of the interviewing, my son Danny for much of the drafting of this manuscript, my husband Steve for editing and guidance throughout the process, and Adam and Sarah for editing. My need for all this help strained the renewed sense of independence I had been building more than I could have imagined, as I was forced to ask more from those close to me than ever before. Having put myself back into a professional context, the anxieties and doubts that made my life as a professor so stressful do creep back in. I wish I'd had more autonomy in writing this book, but I have accepted that this kind of collaboration is what I now need. And there is a joy in it I couldn't have experienced through a solo effort, and deep gratitude for the family dynamic that ultimately made it happen.

• • •

While writing this book, I was frequently asked, "Are you the same person as you were before the stroke?" I often answered that I am partly the same, partly different. This answer is true, but it is not complete because it is not an accurate portrayal of how our identities and lives shift. Nobody has a single, static identity. Our lives are always evolving, and so our identities are always dynamic. Over time, regardless of traumas like stroke, all of us are partly the same, partly different.

I've learned that a stroke doesn't so much strike a blow at a unified whole as it tosses a sharp turn into the gradually sloping path of the narrative we've built over time about where we've been, who we are, and where we're going.

That's jarring, and often painful. But jolted from our cruise-control path, we have the opportunity to choose where we go next. And that can be made, at least in part, into a blessing.

"The most general picture of our essence is an association of drives," philosopher Friedrich Nietzsche wrote. We can use our challenges and the clarity that emerges when we examine them as a lens to make sense of what really matters to us. If we do that, we can choose which drives to pursue and grow and which to ignore. Through this process, we are aligning how we live with who we want to be.

That's why, five years after my stroke, I said, to my own surprise, "I'm a happier person now." I'm certainly not always happier. But friends and colleagues have noticed my disposition has changed in some positive ways. "It's just astounding to me," said Robin Ely. "She smiles now so much more than she did before." As I recover from the stroke, frustrated as I have been, I don't have some of the day-to-day stresses of my old life. Perhaps equally important, I think about stress from a new perspective. Through this experience, I have been able to shape my life more deliberately to reflect what I care about.

I smile and laugh more now, and I am more aware of the dangers of stress and my previous type-A mentality. That does not mean I have left that old me behind completely. Our identities are complex and dynamic. I have evolved, but those desires and fears and old goals are still part of me. I still want to be a mother, a wife, a daughter, a friend, a teacher, an athlete, and much more. How I do those things now is different. How much I do some of those things is also different. But those parts of my identity that were there before the stroke certainly haven't gone anywhere. I've become more aware of what gives my life meaning and the choices I can make. I think I now have more control than before over which aspects of my identity to prioritize. I cherish this perspective, and also know that I can sometimes lose track of it.

That brings me to an insight about myself I gained only while writing this chapter. Throughout my life, I have been on a constant quest for growth. I am not satisfied with what I know now, what I have done so far, how the world works today. I want to make things better, make myself better, and yes, at times prove to others that I am capable of even more. This went too far at times, raising my ambitions and my stress. But seeking new challenges is a core part of who I have been, and who I still am.

I hope this book and the stories told will help many survivors in small ways or large. But to some degree, we each have to learn and grow into important lessons on our own, in our own way. I was a sociologist for twenty-five years, but I had to write this book for five years to come back to an understanding that every Introduction to Psychology professor teaches through Maslow's famous pyramid—that the self-actualization at the top of the pyramid represents our human desire for personal growth. That is what I have truly craved since my stroke. Through the writing of this book, I have learned to obsess less about deficiencies in my basic and psychological needs and focus more on building a fulfilling life that lets me achieve and expand my potential going forward.

CHAPTER 19.

Fulfillment through Growth

During my time in Boston doing the clinical trial for Melodic Intonation Therapy, I stayed for four months with my friend and colleague Robin Ely. She knew me before my stroke as pretty high-strung. "She had even been stressed out the year she was on her sabbatical—supposedly a time for renewal," Robin recalled. She didn't know what to expect when I arrived at her home a year after my stroke to start the program. I surprised her. "She had always been a sort of a glass-half-empty person," Robin said, accurately. "But that completely went away. When she was living with us, she was the happiest I'd ever seen her, laughing all the time—that was the most noticeable thing," she said. Part of it was my encouragement from the therapy and the relief of reclaiming some independence by living in Boston. But it was more than that.

It was my experience of personal growth. In a very meaningful way, my outlook on the world had changed, making me happier and giving me a more positive disposition. For most of my life, my approach to the world had been one of determination and stubborn ambition. Fighting to recover from stroke forced me to slow down and reflect in ways I never had before. I had to choose how to think about my future, and that meant letting go of some ways of being that didn't fit my changing goals.

When I was a professor at Stanford, I often felt like I was a small fish in a very big pond. I felt stressed about my performance, my progression, and my standing in the university. I cared deeply about my profession, but I spent more time and energy comparing myself to the elite group around me than thinking about the intrinsic satisfaction I got from my work. With more distance (and yes, more frustration now), I can see how lucky I was in my position, how much I achieved, but also how narrow my previous perspective was. That lets me look with more appreciation on what I do have now and lets me focus more clearly on ways I can grow to become happier and more fulfilled in the future.

. . .

Recognizing silver linings and opportunities for growth has been one of the primary strategies I have used to make the years of adversity more tolerable and meaningful. Survivors have found new appreciation for family, deeper perspective on their values, and new depths of caring, kindness, and generosity that have enriched their lives as well as the lives of others. This strategy is far more than a way to "make lemonade out of lemons" in times of adversity. It is an extreme case of a fundamental human experience.

Seeking growth through challenge is one of the primary ways people find satisfaction in life. Renowned psychologist Mihály Csíkszentmihályi found that people are most satisfied when their limits are pushed just to the bounds of what they are capable of. In such situations of achievable adversity, people become more complex. They enter what Csíkszentmihályi calls a state of flow: "a mental state of complete absorption in the current experience."[133] Athletes and musicians are often used to exemplify this state, but it can be accessed during work, hobbies, deep conversation, or many other parts of life. In day-to-day activities, when the challenge is very close to current capabilities, flow happens naturally.

In the incredible book *Man's Search for Meaning*, psychiatrist and neurologist Victor Frankl recounts his journey through concentration camps in the Holocaust, and his arrival at logotherapy, based on the premise that finding meaning in life is the most powerful motivating force to humans.[134] In this framework, the quest for meaning and understanding is not just an aspect of our lives; it is central to who we are and who we are becoming.

We are motivated by our many desires and ideas, some of which are aligned and some of which compete.

Faced with a trauma like stroke, the opportunities for both challenge and growth are great. If we look at our challenge as regaining all our previous capabilities, we'll see an overwhelming mountain of adversity and feel ever-mounting frustration. This is why sensemaking, goal setting, and small wins become so important. We can clarify what we value most in life, set goals that will help us meet them, and achieve repeated small wins in pursuit of them. In this way, we can achieve not just recovery, but satisfying growth and fundamental meaning in our lives.

• • •

When I set out to write this book, it was partly to fill a void. My job as a professor had been taken away. My identity had been stolen. My membership in the Stanford community, the tenure that signaled my professional achievement, the vocation of mentoring and teaching students, the calling of creating knowledge that could help others make a difference in their lives and the world—all of these seemed to be gone because my body wasn't capable. My sense of purpose and meaning and self-worth were gone with them. I thought that by writing this book I could reclaim some of that, prove that I could still do it, and yes, prove everyone wrong. I am still me, stubborn and determined. *I am Debra Meyerson.*

That's not at all how writing this book has played out. It has forced me to reflect, to listen to others, and to think deeply about what I really want to share with other survivors. I learned from their stories and from reliving my own. For years, I've been researching, and writing, and reminding myself to take my own advice. It's often hard. My family would often remind me to "practice what I preach." Through this process, I've learned more about how my relationships have changed, why I cared so much about being a professor, and just how lucky I've been to have not only a support network for myself but also a support network for my support network. I've learned more fully who I am. I've become better at setting small goals for myself, at recognizing when I enter a funk, and at figuring out how I need to adjust my perspective when needed. I've learned to better express gratitude, consideration, and vulnerability—and maybe more importantly, to more fully feel them. Yes, I am still Debra Meyerson, but not the same Debra Meyerson.

The stroke knocked me down, and I got back up. But more, I grew up. I didn't grow on my own, just as I am not recovering on my own. Every survivor in this book helped me see new aspects of the journey and inspired me to push further—to think more deeply. All the friends I've mentioned, and many others, have talked me through struggles and challenges and improvements. Every book and article referenced in my research has helped me make sense of what I was learning. *I am Debra Meyerson*, but only because of those around me.

I had advantages in my path to growth: the resources and support to write this book, formal training in sociology to guide my thinking, and an amazing family and other supporters to walk this journey with me. Other survivors in this book had different advantages, different struggles, and different recoveries. Every one of them had to find their own route to rebuilding themselves and finding a fulfilling life, to redefining their own recovery and how it would be a force for growth in the long run.

I think the survivors who are thriving share a few critical things: a dedication to fighting to regain capabilities well beyond twelve months; an outlook driven by building a better future rather than recovering the past; and a commitment to accepting support, setting achievable goals, celebrating small wins and silver linings, and drawing on deeper meaning. They are making a conscious choice to learn from the journey, draw perspective from its challenges, and grow from the experience.

This personal growth does not require huge insights, deep philosophies, or macro views on life. We do not need to define our purpose in this world and how our trauma changed it. We simply need to be aware. In the midst of our frustration during therapy, when do we slip into flow? In times of despair, when do we feel glimmers of lightness and moments of joy? Who makes us feel loved, understood, and good about ourselves? When do we completely forget about our stroke and find ourselves at peace and filled with a sense of purpose? For me, it makes all the difference in the world if I can notice those moments. I think of them like a light bulb turning on over my head, make a small mental note, and then keep living life.

I think everyone has many of these moments and can become better at catching them. The challenges of stroke recovery can become a blessing, as our slower pace and more intentional life make it easier to notice them and, perhaps, pause and think about them. These light bulbs become spotlights on the times we enjoy, the feelings we cherish, the things in our lives we find meaningful. They add up. Soon, we have a pathway lit with our own values, shining the way toward a life that will be meaningful and fulfilling. Then we just have to embrace it and continue carving that path forward.

Our identity is not a static thing. It cannot be taken away from us, nor can we throw it away. It is a mix of our desires and ambitions, our associations and roles, our values and our relationships, and our emotions and our thoughts. These aspects of our life continually interact. They come to the surface or fade into the background, gain momentum, or lose steam. We choose to elevate and build up some parts and hide others, and we construct a narrative for ourselves about who we are. But this winding path is never done. Our primary drivers are never fully clear, even to ourselves; the turns we will take next are never fully determined. Our options may be more limited because we have disabilities, but we still get to choose where we steer our path next, who we become now. Stroke may cripple some of our capabilities, shut down aspects of our life we thought were important, knock us off the direction we thought we were headed. But for those of us lucky enough to be survivors, stroke does not steal our future or who we get to become next.

Acknowledgments

Given how much help I needed to write this book and how many people have helped me recover, this section simply must be long. I am truly blessed to have so many people to thank.

I want to start with a truly special thanks to Sally Collings. For almost three years, Sally, you worked tirelessly with me on this project. From concept, to proposal, to finding an agent, and completing a first draft. You helped make it possible to interview survivors, collect stories, and do critical research, bringing not only your time and expertise but your heart as well— showing genuine interest, empathy, compassion, and caring to me and all of those you met. Were it not for my decision to substantially alter my approach to this book, after you helped create the first draft and had moved on to other projects, you would have been my coauthor. This book would not exist, let alone be what it is, without you.

To each and every survivor who shared your time and stories with candor and often great emotion, thank you. Many of you, like me, have decided to make your story an integral part of your life, and in some cases your work, and are very public about your journeys. Others of you have wished to remain private, and for you I have used a pseudonym throughout the text. Either way, you have all educated me, inspired me, contributed to my journey, and made this book possible. I cannot thank you enough for your contributions to me, this book, and the world in which you live.

I am truly blessed with an incredible family—both the one I chose and helped create, as well as the one into which I was born. The strength and depth of their support—in life and in recovery, not to mention in writing this book—is truly incredible. I hope that my love and appreciation is already clear throughout the pages of this book, but of course I want to acknowledge it here.

Danny—that you are my coauthor really says it all. Three years into this project, with a full draft in hand, you had just turned twenty-eight years old and were between jobs exploring your next professional step. You asked if you could be helpful and the rest, as they say, is history. During our two-week stay at Lake Tahoe, I realized I wanted the book to have a different structure, and you led Dad and me through a process to rough it out. Then you offered to help start the redrafting process. For the next fifteen months—while researching career options, interviewing coast to coast, starting a new job in a new industry that led you back to New York and frequent eighty-hour workweeks, you have been my writing partner. It would have been completely unreasonable for me to ask you to use—I should say create—spare hours and days to keep going and use much of your vacation time to create a few periods of focus. And I didn't ask, because you insisted on doing it. You've put every spare moment into this book—and then some, often to the degree that we worried about you. You never let my frustration with our pace deter you, handling my impatience with a grace and maturity that couldn't make a mother more proud. Your involvement not only was critical to bringing this book to life, it has made the process of writing it something I will treasure forever. Congrats on your first book; I'm guessing it won't be your last.

Adam, while you were the farthest away at the time of my stroke, you were nearest for three years after you graduated. Having you nearby to begin your adulthood and so willing to make Dad and me a big part of your life was such a blessing. When I dropped you off for college just before my stroke, we were in the midst of clichéd parent–adolescent son growing pains. To watch you mature into such a composed, thoughtful, and at times even disciplined man has been one of the great rewards of motherhood. Balancing the role of both peacemaking "middle child" and trouble-causing prankster, your terrible puns and wonderful attitude lift our family from tension to laughter like no one else can.

Sarah, your "puffer face" has regularly helped me out of my bouts with unhealthy intensity and frustration, forcing a smile onto my face when I need it the most. During a challenge like this, I can't overstate the value of your timely "attitude adjustments." But you have done far more than make this journey more bearable; you have at times led the way through it. Danny and I never once made it through an editing round of Chapter 9 without tearing up over your Chapel Talk. You are the youngest in the family but probably the first of us to find meaning and growth from this unwanted journey. You have inspired all of us and become a source of family strength and perspective well ahead of your years.

Adam and Sarah—you both have been critical to this book as well, eagerly helping with research, drafting, editing, and feedback. You've made the book far better, the commitment achievable for Danny and Dad, and the project a full-family endeavor. I love and appreciate you both even more than I knew I could.

Steve—in our twenty-two years of marriage before my stroke, I had learned what a remarkable person, and husband, you are. In 2001, when you read and edited draft after draft of *Tempered Radicals*, I learned how effective you could be in both editing and moral support. Neither prepared me for how amazing you could be through my stroke recovery and, more relevant here, the process of writing this book. You've taken on *Identity Theft* with an incredible depth of heart. Your patience is remarkable; I wish I could model it more myself and have watched in real time as our kids have learned from you. Your unwavering belief that this story needed to be told, and that I could tell it, kept me going. You understood long before I did that the writing process would help my own emotional journey in profound ways; but you were smart enough not to say that until we were well on our way.

Your incredible support in the writing of *Identity Theft* is of course just the tip of the iceberg—you have been by my side every minute of this journey that is our lives. I love you so much.

Mom, you're a rock. Thank you for your strength and support, which has never wavered. I had my stroke when you were already in crisis, and you still dropped everything to support me and my family. You are a model for selfless love. You so often are my voice of hope and persistence when I want to look down; everything I learned about tenacity I learned from you. You've been a constant support through the writing of this book, encouraging me generally, reminding us of stories from our journey, and commenting on drafts along the way. I love you and thank you.

I also want to thank my late dad, Aubrey Meyerson, whom we lost twenty-three years ago when he was in the prime of life. Dad—I would not be who I am without you. I still miss you so very much.

Aaron, thank you for your lifelong support—you are an incredible brother. You have been a constant presence throughout the writing process and before. You and your family have been an outside light, constantly reminding me that the world of people and things I love keeps turning—that my journey is not all there is. And talented as you are, you too have been an "inside" reader of drafts—helping to make this a better book. Thank you, and I love you.

My friends are truly incredible. Robin Ely—you are a special friend. And as a professional colleague and coauthor before, you have a unique perspective on my journey. Just a year after my stroke, you and Harry (and your daughter Francesca, who we now get to claim as a Californian) welcomed me into your home for four months—more generous than I could expect and more helpful than I could have imagined. And you somehow found time to read and comment on a full draft. Molly Stuart, you were there at Renown Hospital in Reno the day after my stroke. I can't tell you how much your presence throughout this journey has meant to me. To my childhood friends, Debbie Steinberg and Debbie Landau—your abilities to make me laugh at any point have kept me sane. And Lizzie Bradley—almost since the day we met in 1986 you have been such a special friend and source of support.

Kim Menninger, Karen Jordan, and Beth Cross—my other local "go to" companions and dear friends throughout this journey—I couldn't have done it without you. Somehow, you all make time for me when it counts the most, despite your crazy schedules. To the "La Entrada Ladies"—you know who you are. My growing connection with you all—old friends and new ones alike—has meant so much to me. And of course, my women's support group since 1983—Amy Beringer, Patty Collier, Lisa Kelley, Patty Jackson, Ann Mathieson, Sue Panella, Su-Moon Paik, and Nancy Ryan—a source of constant support of course, you also provided that critical nudge when I first thought about writing this book. Debbie Kolb, always a dear friend and colleague, you were so important to me during my first real test of independence when I was in Boston. Joanne Martin—from advisor, to mentor, to colleague and friend. Even from retirement in Hawaii, you find ways to support me. Thank you all so very much.

As much as my support network has been critical, so has Steve's—I am completely aware he could not do for me what he does, be who he is, without them. To Tony Stayner, Steve's "go to" and simply incredible friend of more than thirty years. And Kevin Menninger, his increasingly important neighborhood buddy. To his version of my Stanford Business School-rooted support group—Tony, Howie Rosen, Ken Kelley, Bill Shott, and Paul Perez—gathering "semi-consistently" since graduation for birthdays, burgers, and beers at the Dutch Goose—where Steve could both escape the stress of stroke recovery and talk about it, from the earliest months after my stroke. To his long-distance regulars from his undergrad days, always up for a commute-time phone call—Jodi Kravitz and Teddy Berenblum—as well as Drew Lieberman more locally, with whom he could grab a coffee, a run, or a walk.

I know how important you all are to Steve, and how much you helped him through his part of this journey.

And thanks to those of you who engineered some particularly "cathartic" events for Steve—most notably his first boys' ski getaway when Drew Dougherty, Tony, and Kevin "hijacked" Steve about six months after my stroke when you knew he needed an escape. You and others helped Steve learn what he needed to "stay sane" during this journey. To Martin Eakes and all of Steve's colleagues at Self-Help—you are all truly amazing for the work you do and the work culture you have created. I'm not sure Steve could have done what he's done for me if he worked anyplace else. And of course, to Steve's family—mother Marjorie, late father George, and sister Marcia—for being Steve's constant and critical support throughout this journey, and always.

Thank you to the incredible people who were directly involved in helping me. There are hundreds of you who have helped my long and complicated journey, so please know I thank you even if you are not mentioned specifically. Dr. Chitra Venkatasubramanian (try saying that with aphasia!), aka Dr. Venkat—you "adopted" me as your long-term neurology patient when I graduated from the collective care of the Stroke Group at Stanford Hospital—I can't tell you how glad I am that you did. Dr. Sarah Watson, my primary care physician, you make time for me whenever I need it. And you are both so supportive of creative and nontraditional care in the evolving world of stroke recovery.

To Waleed Al-Oboudi, you have guided my physical and occupational therapy work since almost the beginning and I can't thank you—and many you have trained, including Amelia Chang, Rudy Flores, Ryan Carmona, Dan Densley, Trudy Maaskant, Sarah Williams, Pam Hansenium, and Carrie Sullivan—enough. And Diane Pacholski, thank you for getting me started in therapy and referring me to Waleed when my work at Stanford was complete. Also, Jennifer Williams, who has worked with me through the stem cell trial at Stanford.

Regaining speech has been such a critical part of my recovery, and there are so many who have helped. My sincere thanks to Megan DePuy and Kelly Crisp for working with me so patiently in those early months at the Stanford outpatient program, and to Andrea Norton who led my Melodic Intonation Therapy—for four months of intensive work in Boston. To Leora Cherney, director of the intensive aphasia program at Shirley Ryan AbilityLab, which I have done twice, and the fantastic team you assemble for that program. And finally, to Lisa Levine-Sporer, for leading my ongoing work these past five years—I can't thank you enough for your countless hours of therapy, guidance . . . and friendship.

Once I started down the path of writing this book, it became clear that I would use it as a foundation for advocacy and education—that I want to build a community around this work. That led me to create a website and social media presence, something I could not do on my own. Thank you, Rebecca Mayer, Madeleine Fawcett, Megan De Tranc, Ellie Frymire, and now Jennifer Moilanen-Harper for leading this work. And Jane Evered, who did critical research early on.

And finally, people beyond my family who have been intimately involved in the actual writing of this book.

To our team of "nonprofessional" but extremely expert readers who made time in your busy lives to fit into our compressed schedule as we neared the end. I thanked you, Robin and Aaron, above, and along with Jose Riera, Jodi Kravitz, and Marcia Zuckerman, you gave us incredible input that profoundly influenced this book. I can't thank you enough. And thanks to Steve Goodman and Ruth Levine, whose creativity during an enjoyable dinner led to the title for this book.

And finally, our team of professionals at Andrews McMeel. Thank you, Andy Sareyan, for suggesting to Steve that this would be a book your team might like to bring to life. To Kirsty Melville—your immediate enthusiasm was incredible, and we knew immediately that you really understood what

I was trying to do, something missed by so many others. Jean Lucas—you have made the complex process of getting this over the finish line and into the hands of readers understandable and less intimidating. And Chris Schillig—you have given us invaluable help through your early directional guidance to your detailed and exceptional editing as we approached our final manuscript. Thanks to you all.

Survivor Biographies

Below are brief biographies of twenty-five incredible people who gave time and energy, often along with a partner, child, parent, or caregiver, to tell a bit of their story to help create this book. I am both appreciative and humbled by what they have shared. My goal was to include a very broad perspective in this book—every person is different, every stroke is different, every recovery is different. I hoped that by bringing both my own experiences, as well as those from a diverse group of survivors—or as Kathy Howard might say, Thrivers—I could write a book that might support all survivors in some meaningful way.

Included in this group are people of many races, ethnicities, and countries of origin. Of course, there are both men and women (no one who is gender fluid as far as I know.) People in this group suffered their stroke or other health trauma from the age of thirteen at the youngest to sixty-four at the oldest. They were as little as one year beyond their stroke and as much as nineteen years. All of them had significant disabilities immediately following their strokes, and all have at least some that continue to impact their lives. For a few, these are minor, but most continue to have meaningful physical, speech, or other disabilities. One survivor has locked-in syndrome and is paralyzed from the neck down with no ability to speak at all. They all live in the United States, across the map from Boston to St. Louis to California.

For each of us, this is a very personal journey. In many cases, people have shared very personal, even intimate, thoughts. I cannot thank you all enough. Several people have chosen to keep their identities anonymous, and in those cases, I have used a pseudonym throughout the book, including below. For many, they have shared their names, and these are used throughout.

I hope these brief biographies serve as a useful resource. When you come across an example in the book where a person is not fully described, it might be helpful to remind yourself about his or her basic story. And reading them through, from start to finish, might also be useful. These are all incredible people who are on heroic journeys. As I did, you may see bits and pieces of yourself or your loved ones in many of them. I find their stories both informative and inspiring. I hope you will as well.

JOSÉ COFIÑO

José Cofiño was born in Cuba, but his family left everything behind in 1959 to escape the revolution and migrate to Mexico City. Things there were tough—his father passed away when José was six, and his brother was killed riding a bike a year later. In 1969, José and his mom rode a bus for four days to a new home in Washington, DC, where things got better. José received scholarships to attend religious schools through high school, graduated from George Washington University, and then later Stanford Business School, where he met my husband Steve. He excelled professionally with managerial roles at companies like Disney and PepsiCo. But José was also living with a secret; he struggled with his identity, specifically his sexuality. Worried that family and friends might not approve, he didn't come out until he was in his thirties. He shouldn't have worried—the embrace he received was incredible.

In 2012, just after his twenty-fifth business school reunion, José was diagnosed with ALS. It took him and his partner Ben Trust about a year to get over the shock and to figure out how best to tell his mom. But his prior experience made it clear to him he could get strength from and give strength to others, if he was open about his battle with ALS. José and Ben rearranged their lives to accomplish two goals: live life as fully as they could while they still had time together; and make a difference by raising awareness about ALS and raising money to help find a cure. In 2014, they founded Beyond ALS (https://www.beyondals.org/) to do the latter. José passed away in October 2017. He struggled with his changing identity as ALS robbed him of motor function, but far less than many as he quickly acknowledged his condition and did the best he could with it, openly and vigorously. We thank José and Ben for spending time with us so close to the end of their journey together.

CAM COMPTON

In early 2012, Cam Compton was fifty-two years old, living in her hometown of St. Louis, Missouri, around the corner from her parents, and she was adjusting to change—she had gotten divorced the year before. She was not only learning to be a single mom to her sixteen-year-old daughter, she was also caring for her older daughter's child, who was ten years old. Cam's financial situation wasn't flush, but it was stable. She had a good job as a medical secretary at Mercy Medical Center, where she had worked for thirty years, and she was managing to raise two kids, make payments on a modest home, and live a comfortable life. Cam was always busy. In addition to full-time work, she took her two kids to lots of sports and other activities, ran two Girl Scout troops, was a room parent, and volunteered at a homeless shelter at her church. Her stroke in March 2012 changed all that.

Initially unable to walk at all, Cam left the rehab hospital using a walker. She still walks with a limp, has significant weakness in one arm, and suffers from balance problems. Her memory and cognitive functions still aren't what they used to be. She was able to return to work but can only work twenty-four hours a week more than six years after her stroke. Less income and significant medical expenses put Cam in a very tough financial situation, peaking five years after her stroke when her long-term disability insurance company just stopped making payments. They told her she no longer had a disability and could go back to work full time.

With the help of a lawyer, she finally got her benefits back. Through all these challenges, Cam maintained a fantastically upbeat attitude. She talks passionately about the importance of finding purpose, and she now finds hers helping other stroke survivors. Cam leads a stroke support group that meets twice a month, started a Junk in your Trunk mobile garage sale to benefit stroke efforts, and does a stroke segment for a podcast called Hand in Hand. And always open to new possibilities, she tells me, "I met a wonderful man named Joe; he loves me for who I am, brain injury and all." They got married in April 2018.

ISAIAH CUSTODIO

Isaiah Custodio is the youngest survivor I talked to for this book, about a year after an arteriovenous malformation (AVM) caused massive bleeding in his brain when he was just thirteen years old. He was at football practice in his hometown of Greenville, South Carolina, when he told his coach he had a headache. He asked if he could sit for a minute, jogged to the fence, collapsed, threw up twice, and could only say, "Help. Home." They put him in a car, where he immediately passed out. Raised in a religious family, Isaiah later said, "I saw two angels, right then and there."

The surgeon told his family that he would try to stop the bleeding with emergency surgery, but they should be prepared for the worst. Thankfully, the surgery went well, and a year after his stroke, Isaiah was working hard on therapy. He had regained most of his speech ability and was walking pretty well, albeit with a limp. Vision, memory, and concentration were his biggest challenges. Isaiah's mom talked excitedly of his progress and her hopes that he continues to improve, so he can regain his amazing smile (hurt by lip droop) and his love of reading (he used to read a four-hundred-page book in a day). Isaiah talked about missing sports. But they both were clear that they saw a great future for Isaiah no matter what disabilities remain.

MARK DAVIS

A self-proclaimed workaholic, Mark started working at odd jobs as a kid, joined UPS when he was twenty, and always had other work going on the side. He had saved enough money over the years to buy six rental properties around the Bay Area. He was very proud of the life he had built. "I thought I did pretty good for myself," he shared, but he did say he regrets that he never got married or had kids. At age fifty-two, he had a severe stroke that forced him to do something he hadn't done since he was a teenager—stop working. He retired from UPS after thirty-two years; when I met him five years later, he was spending most of his time managing his rental properties. His stroke forced him to slow down and reflect on his life in a way that his consistent sixty- to one-hundred-hour workweeks never allowed him to do. "I feel like life, the universe, or whatever sits you down does it for a reason," he told me.

Many people I met while writing this book turned to their faith for a sense of meaning after their stroke. Mark did something a bit different. He didn't reject it, but he used his newfound time to understand it better. Mark was always inquisitive and questioning, but the religion he grew up with taught him to accept certain things as fact. As he dug deeper, he disconnected somewhat from the church, but he found a new passion in learning about his African-American heritage. That has been incredibly fulfilling and given him a better connection to his identity. Understanding this history has given him a more holistic view of himself and his place in the world, for which he largely credits his stroke.

JULIA FOX GARRISON

Julia Fox Garrison grew up with eight brothers in a tight-knit family in Andover, Massachusetts. In 1997, at age thirty-seven, Julia was living north of Boston with her husband Jim and three-year-old son Rory, and she had a massive hemorrhage that caused a paralyzing stroke. Her left side was completely immobile, and she needed help with everything. Her doctors told her she was lucky to be alive and that, if she survived, she shouldn't expect to walk again. For twenty years, Julia has proven most of the doubters wrong. Although she still walks with a brace on her leg and uses a cane for support (the same one they gave her when she first escaped her wheelchair), she has regained her independence and has consciously reshaped her life.

Before her stroke, in addition to her roles as mother and wife, Julia was a manager at a software company on the fast track to directorship. Much of her life revolved around her work—her friends were from the company, and she even met her husband Jim at a prior job. Julia was not able to return to her position at the software company, but she would be the first to tell you that was a blessing in disguise. She made a deliberate decision to redirect her life and became a writer, health-care advocate, and motivational speaker. In 2006, HarperCollins Publishers released her memoir entitled *Don't Leave Me This Way: Or When I Get Back on My Feet You'll Be Sorry*. Her book, a two-time *Boston Globe* bestseller, is described as "funny, touching, and profoundly moving," as she takes on an entrenched medical community "with wit and grit," challenging doctors to remember that all patients are human beings and that encouragement and optimism are critical to the path of recovery. (www.juliafoxgarrison.com)

EMMANUEL "MANNY" GIGANTE

In 2003, Manny Gigante was a twenty-nine-year-old network engineer living with his wife, two daughters, and a son in San Jose, California. Manny was born to Filipino immigrant parents and was working very hard to fulfill the vision that brings so many immigrants to America—creating a better life for himself, his family, and future generations. Of course, he was trying to be a good husband and father, but most of his time and energy were focused on professional advancement and making as much money as possible as quickly as possible. Then out of nowhere, Manny suffered a massive stroke. It left him in a wheelchair for more than two years and with substantial ongoing physical disabilities even fifteen years later. He is grateful that his stroke didn't rob him of his speech and cognitive abilities.

Manny struggled to reconcile his life as a person with disabilities with how he envisioned his role as a man, husband, and father. Two years after his stroke, his crisis became worse when his first son was killed in an accident. He wondered constantly if his disabilities had contributed to that outcome. His culture told him a man should be strong, a protector, a provider—macho, he explained—traits he no longer possessed, given his physical disabilities. He was thrilled that he and his wife had another son later, but he still felt that his role should be to wrestle with the boy and play catch. Over time, he has revised his beliefs about what it means to be a good father, husband, and man. Manny watched his oldest daughter develop empathy and choose to be an occupational therapist based on his experience. His disabilities forced him out of his prior role as a network engineer, which required physical tasks such as climbing towers. He made a decision to rebuild his life around capabilities he does have, and now has a rewarding career in real estate. Surrounded by family, working a stable job, and with realigned priorities, Manny is far from 100 percent physically, but he says he is living a happy, healthy, and fulfilling life.

TRISH HAMBRIDGE

Trish Hambridge was forty-three in 2008 when she suffered a severe left-brain ischemic stroke. A project manager at Apple, Trish's stroke left her with severe aphasia and motor disability. Before her stroke, Trish drew her energy from sports and her social life. She had been an avid soccer and softball player and an active golfer. She had a magnetic personality that drew people in, and she thrived in social situations. Her friends describe her as always being the jokester in the room. Since her stroke, she has found ways to communicate and engage with the community that help her nourish her love of human connection. She also works with the Aphasia Recovery Connection and the Bay Area Aphasia Circle to engage with people she can more easily communicate with.

Since her stroke, Trish has maintained her core personality. She golfs with a one-handed club and has some preprogrammed one-liners in her iPad that help her come up with a good punch line when needed. Trish recently moved to Florida to save money. Still unable to work, she lives on disability and spends her time working toward recovery and engaging with the stroke community. She has family spread across the country: a brother in Seattle, parents in Niagara, and a sister in New York. Traveling to visit them allows her to indulge her love of adventure. She still works tirelessly at therapy and is seeing improvements in her speech all the time.

WHITNEY HARDY

I've known Whitney Hardy since she was born in Truckee, California, to two of my closest friends, Molly Stuart and Tony Hardy. As a four-month-old, she amused our mostly single, childless friends the night before my wedding to Steve by rolling over on a hotel bed for the very first time. She was an active kid in the mountains—skiing in the winter and playing competitive soccer in spring, summer, and fall. In 2010, she graduated from Tufts University in Boston, where she played four years of varsity soccer. She remained in Boston to work for a real estate investment firm and became engaged to her college boyfriend in 2014. Two months later, out for a winter run, she was hit by a car. Her leg was shattered and, even more devastating, she suffered severe traumatic brain injury.

Her journey since then has been tough. First, she battled for her life, having several brain operations, and spent months in hospitals. Then came several years of intensive therapy. Her major disabilities now involve loss of memory and processing skills. As she improved, she and her fiancé, who had been more of a partner in recovery than anyone could have expected, began talking about wedding plans. But in the end, he just couldn't go through with it. As much as he still loved her, he was unable to start their life together when she couldn't be a full emotional partner. Whitney returned to Truckee and is again living with her parents. She is gaining more independence as time passes, including driving. She has done some soccer coaching and has had some success with modest jobs. Whitney and her parents have had to rethink their futures in ways they never expected. But they are moving forward, and Whitney continues to build a new life around her slowly improving capabilities.

ANDREA HELFT

At forty-four, Andrea Helft was living a life familiar to many professional women in Palo Alto, California. She was working long hours as a cofounder of a small online retail business and also as a business consultant. She juggled that with her roles as mother of three young children, wife of a husband also working in a demanding job, and avid recreational athlete with a special focus on running. That life came to a halt when she suffered a severe hemorrhagic stroke. Although she had some physical disabilities for a while after her stroke—weakness in her right arm and loss of balance—the most debilitating impact of Andrea's stroke was extreme fatigue and loss of memory. Even after months of recovery and speech therapy, she couldn't remember what question someone asked her even as she was trying to form an answer.

Possibly more than any other survivor I've met, Andrea has embraced her silver linings. Trying to help her rebuild her sense of self, several of her friends joined her on a journey of self-discovery. They are closer than ever, and all have a better sense of what's really important to them. Andrea was able to return to work, but she is less focused on that part of her life and more on family and close friends, giving her what she called "a ball of warmth." She talks about being happier and healthier after her stroke, and she feels that in many ways she is a better person. She isn't alone in finding things that are better after stroke, and she went so far as to say, "I might even do it again if I had to—isn't that crazy?"

KATHY HOWARD

Kathy Howard is a proud, lifelong resident of St. Louis, Missouri. She and her husband Jim worked hard to build a comfortable life and save enough to send their son and daughter to college. Over the years, Kathy worked for the Department of Justice, was a middle school teacher, and then became office manager of an outpatient therapy office. After celebrating her thirty-first wedding anniversary in 2008 when she was fifty-five years old, she was on her way to the couch after dinner when, "It was almost like a zipper was installed here," she points to her back. "I just felt this *wjjjjjt* right to the top of my head." She saw a big black hole in the TV screen, got sick, and everything turned red and green. She didn't know it yet, but she had just had a massive stroke.

Like everyone I've talked to for this book, Kathy had to work hard to get back some of the most basic capabilities. She couldn't walk. She couldn't sit up. But she got motivated. "This feisty little eighty-three-year-old walks into my room with her hand on her hip and said, 'I had a stroke three weeks ago, and I'm walking out of here.' I thought that if she could do that, I could, too. OK, I am just going to fight like a crazy woman." Kathy has done just that, but she also decided that helping and motivating others, like that eighty-three-year old did for her, would become her life's mission. She visits new survivors whenever she can. She started a conversation group called Coffee Cafe-sia for people with aphasia (communication challenge). She founded ABC Stroke Brigade to organize events like the 5K Stampede for Stroke walk/run to support survivors and raise awareness. She hopes to create a therapeutic center that creates recovery opportunities and community when other resources dry up. Despite her disabilities, Kathy is more healthy and fit than before her stroke. She wears a bracelet that says, "Thriving is Surviving," and said that her stroke helped her find her dream job of helping other "Thrivers."

JIM INDELICATO

Jim Indelicato has been dubbed "the marathon man" by his family—he has completed thirty-two of them. He spent forty years in the U.S. Air Force and Air National Guard, in charge of physical fitness for the latter. He has been married to his wife, Diane, for forty-seven years, and they have been best friends since he was fifteen and she was twelve. Together they have raised a son, Jimmy, and two daughters, Joy and Jody. They all live in St. Louis. Also a lifelong fixer, Jim was planning to start a home-rehabbing business in retirement; that plan was cut short by a massive brain stem stroke in September 2010, when he was just fifty-nine years old.

Jim is a workhorse. Despite the extreme severity of his stroke, he was committed from the start to regain all he could. He insisted on wearing track shorts in the hospital. When he got out, he went to therapy twice as long as recommended. He was determined to move from a wheelchair to a walker, which he did in two years, even though he had a trach (breathing tube) in his neck. He got speech therapists to work overtime to help him relearn to swallow; he successfully got rid of the trach and finally enjoyed his first solid meal four years after his stroke. The recovery that Jim, Diane, and the kids dedicated themselves to has inspired many others on their difficult journeys. The range of his activities may have changed, but it's clear that Jim has found ways to continue living the values that drove him his whole life: persistence, discipline, the importance of family, and leadership by example.

MARY JONES

I met Mary Jones in St. Louis in 2016, where she lived alone. But ten years earlier, in 2006, she was living happily in Washington, DC, forty-four years old, married, working as a federal government contractor, with no children. She called her two bichon frise dogs her kids, and they occupied much of her free time. She also loved being surrounded by the history and culture of DC, and took frequent trips to the mountains and beaches nearby.

In April 2006, Mary was at home when she had a severe headache and called 911. She has no memory of what happened next, but she learned later that a blood clot had caused a severe stroke. She spent almost a month in a hospital and rehab facility before returning home, still almost completely immobile.

For about three years, Mary's husband and a paid caretaker met her needs, including changing her diapers while she was bedridden for several months. She did make progress, regaining quite a bit of her mobility, but her husband was worn out. "He called my family in St. Louis and said, 'I'm too tired. I'm done with this. I'm packing up all Mary's stuff, filing for a divorce, and sending her to St. Louis. You guys take care of her.'" Her family decided to place her in what amounted to a nursing home. She hated it but endured. After three years, she decided she could live safely on her own and save her money for more important things, and she moved into a modest apartment. Regaining independence was a huge boost for her both mentally (she had to think for herself) and emotionally. She began finding ways to exercise and do self-therapy—mostly walking for strength and playing memory games on the computer. And she has built community and a social life mostly through church. Despite the loss of active support from family, she is remarkably positive and forward looking and has taken incredible steps to rebuild her life.

CINDY LOPEZ

Cindy Lopez is a vibrant woman with a dazzling smile. In 2014, she was thirty-six and living in Cambridge, Massachusetts, with her husband, a former policeman still working in law enforcement. They had moved from Chicago just a couple of years before, and most of Cindy's family, of Filipino descent, lived in the Midwest. Cindy was working as a grants manager, and life was good for the young couple. Then Cindy had a stroke.

She describes herself as lucky in that she had just been driving around doing errands but had gotten home when it hit. Her husband was also at home and, given his background, saw the signs of stroke immediately and knew to call 911. Cindy is fortunate that she regained enough of her capability to return to her prior job, and that the policies and benefits at her employer really helped make that possible. She explained that she got through the "why me" stage pretty fast. About a decade before, her husband was diagnosed with an incurable illness that could potentially lead to blindness, so she had been through it once before. But Cindy struggled and was still struggling when we spoke, reconciling her sense of identity with the new, less capable body that prevented her from doing so much of what she used to do. She was getting professional support to help figure that out, and she definitely saw herself as being on a journey.

SEAN MALONEY

Sean Maloney grew up in a working-class family and made his way up the corporate ladder over a thirty-one-year career at tech giant Intel. In 2010, he was considered by many to be the anointed one, next in line for CEO; then he had a stroke. He was initially left completely speechless with no mobility on his entire right side. Before his stroke, he was a respected leader in the tech community, and according to his speech therapist, he was a true orator. That was all taken from him when his carotid artery abruptly shut in 2010. With his characteristic determination, he set out to regain as much as he could but found this to be a truly daunting task. "When you learn to speak again, it is the most difficult experience that you've ever had. Running an organization with fifteen thousand people is nothing compared to that. It's mind-blowing."

Like many others I have met, Sean demonstrates tremendous persistence, positive thinking, and a little bit of well-placed stubbornness. And in the nine years since his stroke, he has made incredible recoveries in both his physical and speech capabilities. He, like me and many others, has seized an unexpected silver lining—redirecting his career toward helping the stroke community that he unfortunately joined as a survivor. He has launched efforts to improve awareness (including a bike ride across America) and to develop medical technologies that will help prevent strokes in the future. Sean also spoke powerfully and gratefully about his deepened relationship with his wife and children. When asked whether he would go back to his old life if he had the choice, he reflexively responded, "Of course I would." He hesitated, then continued, "I don't know. Half of me would, half of me wouldn't."

MICHAEL MCDERMOTT

Michael McDermott considers himself to be a lucky survivor on many fronts. While driving through Ohio on a sales trip for his employer of twenty-five years, Michael had a stroke. He tried to drive back to his hotel, falling asleep at the wheel multiple times and scraping against the guardrail. Then he passed out in his car for almost twenty-four hours after he somehow made it back to the hotel. And yet, once he was finally found and taken to the hospital, he was able to regain much of his physical and speech ability within a week and most of the rest after a few months of therapy. He knows just how lucky he is—to be alive, to have made a substantial physical recovery, and to have somehow avoided injuring others during that fateful drive back to his hotel.

Lucky, yes, but not easy. Divorced and living in Ohio, Michael went back to work, confident that the minor lingering effects of his stroke wouldn't interfere with doing his job. Not only didn't his employer try to make small accommodations but they also expanded the scope of his job, including even greater travel requirements. Michael was concerned that it would be too much and, having worked there twenty-five years, decided to be upfront about it. He was fired. In his early sixties, Michael has been unable to find another job. So he retired early and is making ends meet with a combination of savings, a small pension, and Social Security—a far cry from his prior almost six-figure income. Michael now talks with other stroke survivors whenever he can. He knows that compared with many, he got off easy, but his stroke has changed the course of his life dramatically.

RANDY MILLER

After suffering a stroke at age fifty-one, in the prime of his career as an IT manager in St. Louis, Missouri, Randy Miller was left with an unusual form of aphasia. Unable to process his own speech, Randy is constantly questioning the words that come out of his mouth. The result is rough, choppy sentences that can be hard to follow. His hearing is intact, as is his cognitive processing, but the disconnect between what he is thinking and the words that he says makes speech extremely difficult. Unable to return to work, Randy now spends most of his time doing speech therapy through various programs or on his own. Like many married survivors, Randy's stroke has had an almost equally severe impact on the life of his wife Rose, who took early retirement to help care for him. The stroke flipped their life upside down, with both suffering some intermittent depression as a result. But they have also found ways to become closer and enjoy a deeper relationship with each other.

Following the stroke, many friendships were tested, especially those related to work activities. But the strongest ones survived, even deepened, and they developed new close friends from their work in the survivor community, especially the weekly aphasia meet-up group they started. Initially, they tended to socialize with old friends or new friends separately. Then the groups started to mix, which has really enriched their lives. And though their kids are in college out of state, the stroke has brought them new appreciation for the time the family can spend together. Despite the many difficult challenges resulting from the stroke, new and stronger relationships have clearly brought some silver linings to Randy and Rose.

ROCIO ROJAS

Just two weeks after giving birth to her first child, Rocio was getting out of bed when she felt a sudden pain and then passed out. At age thirty-two, Rocio had a stroke. Initially, her speech and physical abilities were severely affected, and after maternity leave, she could not return to her job as a call center supervisor. Living in Riverbank, California, she had great support from her family, many of whom lived nearby. They were particularly helpful at night during that first year, as her husband's job involved working night shifts. She is also glad that in preparation for having their first child, Rocio and her husband had cut back and repaid some debt. That made the financial hit from medical expenses and her not going back to work a bit easier.

Rocio is one of the luckier survivors I've spoken to, with speech and many of her physical capabilities returning quite well within a few years. But she still has difficulties with tasks that used to be easy—some because of lost dexterity and some because her brain just doesn't seem to work as quickly. Rocio shared that she could not help but think, "I'm freaking thirty-two, this really had to happen to me?" But she also knows how much worse it could have been and generally keeps a positive, forward-looking mindset.

GAIL RUSCH

Gail Rusch grew up near Chicago, Illinois, then moved to La Quinta, California, in her early twenties when her ex-husband was transferred there with the U. S. Navy. She moved to San Francisco in her midthirties shortly after a divorce. When I met her in 2016, she was living in San Pablo, California, and it had been fourteen years since the stroke she suffered in 2002, when she was fifty-three. As a single, African-American mother with two children to support, she started working after her divorce as a customer-service trainer at a telecom company. Then she had a series of positions at Federal Express—loading packages, secretarial work, administrative assistant, and eventually training again. She did the AIDS Walk San Francisco every year, and one year got inspired by posters to train for the Hawaii Marathon. She had never run before, but she completed the race. Through these activities, someone recognized her natural training skills, and she was asked to be a weekend coach for the AIDS organization, helping other runners train for marathons. Her children were living in California and Montana when she had her stroke, and she had been with her sweetheart for fifteen years—now her partner for more than thirty years—though she never wanted to remarry.

Like many other survivors, Gail initially lost the use of one side of her body. She still has to cook with one hand (she loves her one-handed chopper!) and walks with some difficulty. She was not able to return to work, and for a while was stuck asking the proverbial, "Why me?" With support from her partner, kids, and friends, she escaped that mindset and decided to rebuild herself from the inside out. In her late fifties, she enrolled at Alameda Junior College and after two successful years she was accepted to Cal State University. She overcame ongoing speech challenges and significant physical disabilities, as well as a two-year bout with cancer that she seems to have won. In 2016, after nine years and at the age of sixty-seven, she received her bachelor's degree in human development and family studies. "I think I went to school so I could again really help people. Now I can help kids."

ANTHONY SANTOS

Anthony Santos was twenty-two years old when I met him, three years after he suffered a severe stroke in the summer of 2013. At age nineteen, he had a major concussion, and he stroked from a complication during the resulting brain surgery. The son of Mexican immigrants living in Fremont, California, his mother described him as a kid who loved everything that had to do with sports. Confined to a wheelchair for months after his stroke, he was determined to regain his abilities and return to at least some of the activities he missed so much.

Four years after his stroke, he had regained significant capabilities, and he was quick to tell me that much of his progress came long after the twelve-month mark when his insurance company tried to stop coverage because they said he would not improve further. He fought hard with his insurance provider and won some additional coverage, though not as much as he wanted. We last spoke almost five years after his stroke, and Anthony was still working hard to regain more capabilities, trying to do more and more with his affected left arm and leg. In the years immediately following his stroke, his sole focus was regaining his lost capabilities, but now he balances that with school work (he is back to pursuing a bachelor's degree and a career in nursing) and doing the activities he enjoys most like hiking, tennis, and wakeboarding. While he is still far from his full former capabilities, he has realized the importance and value of living his life as best he can while still working to regain more.

AHAANA SINGH

Ahaana Singh has a history of mental illness, personally and in her family, and she has been diagnosed as mildly bipolar. She believes that complications from her medications caused her hemorrhagic stroke when she was thirty-seven years old. Initially, she was left completely paralyzed on her right side, but she has since regained almost all of her physical abilities. Despite her substantial physical recovery, she has remaining cognitive difficulties, which she calls brain hiccups—she just can't process instructions and other interactions as well as she used to and misses things.

Of Indian descent, living in St. Louis, Missouri, Ahaana is married with no children. She is close to her sister, who provided good support following her stroke, though her difficult relationship with her mom made things harder. Ahaana was a pharmaceutical regulatory affairs professional before her stroke, but she now works part-time in retail because she just can't keep up with the mental demands of her old job. She is thankful she has regained most of her physical abilities, but she finds it can be a curse in disguise. Most people do not realize that she had a stroke, and those who do think she is over it. Because her disabilities are not readily visible, people—even those who were close friends before the stroke—are less patient and understanding than they seem to be with other stroke survivors. Another challenge for her is that she suffers from survivor guilt—knowing how much more she has recovered than many other survivors.

MALIK THOMA

Raised Muslim as the son of Indian immigrants, Malik Thoma was living the American dream in Arizona. Wanting to make a difference, he left a comfortable, well-paying job to start a chain of day spas that trained and hired battered women, giving them a stable job away from their abuser. He had four stores with plans in motion to expand to seven more. He was married with two kids, very busy, taking care of his family and, he thought, poised to make the world a better place through his work. He was physically fit, athletic, and very active. On the way to the hospital for a routine blood test to monitor a congenital health condition, he got a call from a homeless man he had previously befriended. In the middle of a detour to go help him out, Malik suffered a massive stroke.

Malik survived some very threatening medical scares, but like many other survivors of severe strokes, he lost significant functionality on his left side—both his arm and his leg. Like many I've met, he has worked incredibly hard to regain his capabilities and has made significant progress. But compared with many others, he has had a much more difficult time rebuilding his life. The stroke amplified stress that already existed with his wife and other members of his family. Relationships have been damaged and are very tense. He continuously compares his life—and himself—after stroke only with his life and self before stroke, without looking forward. He has had a harder time than most to see the good things still around him and to discover new opportunities.

MARTINA VARNADO

Martina Varnado was diagnosed with multiple sclerosis in 2001. There were no visible symptoms until 2009, and since then, the progression has been relatively slow but steady—from minor loss of motor control, to using a cane for walking, then a walker, and finally using a motorized wheelchair beginning about five years ago. When we last spoke, her speech was not affected at all. Despite her increasing physical disability, she is still working full time as a director in the Office of the Commissioner for the Food and Drug Administration. Martina lives with her husband Art in Baltimore, Maryland; their two daughters are in college, and their son has graduated and lives and works in Arizona.

An ambitious African-American woman, Martina has always been fiercely independent and committed to being a great role model, particularly for her daughters. For her that has meant, among other things, doing as well as she can in her chosen career, maintaining a strong partnership with Art at home, and being there for family and friends whenever needed. She struggles with the fact that it becomes more and more difficult to maintain those three ideals as her MS continues to attack her physical capabilities. She knows she has to renegotiate what success looks like in each of those domains but doesn't want to let go of what it meant for most of her life.

LAURE WANG

Laure Wang is the most physically handicapped survivor I have spoken with. In 2010, when she lived in Hong Kong, she suffered a severe brain-stem stroke that left her, at thirty-nine, with locked-in syndrome—aware and awake but unable to move anything but her eyes. She is a mute quadriplegic. This was a catastrophic event in what had been, or at least looked like, a charmed life. Laure was born in 1971 in Kingston, New York, to Chinese parents. She worked hard, went to Stanford University and Harvard Business School, and worked for blue chip companies like Goldman

Sachs. She cofounded her own private equity firm, Asset Alternatives, with offices in Hong Kong, Beijing, Shanghai, and San Francisco. She married her best friend and had two beautiful sons. And then the stroke.

Devastating? Yes. But a beginning as well. Laure threw herself into therapy. Most notably, she learned to use a technology that would let her write; she can blink her eyes to indicate one letter at a time that shows up on a screen before her. She has written four books. I was particularly moved by *Reflections on A Changed Life* and *Choppy Waters*, a book containing a series of journal entries from 2001 to 2005. She added one more entry, dated January 14, 2017, that says so much about Laure: "I am now turning forty-six years old. I am married to Kabir and have two sons, Marat and Madyn. I am mute and paralyzed from the neck down and, as a result, I communicate solely through blinking. As I read through my old journals, I see a healthy person, physically, but an angst-ridden and unhealthy person, mentally. Today, I might be physically limited, but I know and accept myself. My sailboat might have hit a sandbar, but I won't give up my journey."

DEIDRE "DEE DEE" WARREN

In 2013, Deidre Warren was sixty-four and in the final years of a long career as a registered nurse at a cardiac rehabilitation hospital. A stroke literally knocked her down in the street outside her church. She lived in Millbrae, California, with Mike, her husband of forty-four years, who had retired just six months before her stroke. They have two grown sons who both served in the U.S. Air Force. They are a very close family and big users of facetime and Skype, so they can stay connected even when thousands of miles apart. Even though she was extremely healthy, Deidre told me she wasn't really surprised she had a stroke. Her mother had died from one, and she just thought it might happen to her as well.

When we met two years after her stroke, Deidre was continuing to work hard on therapy but still had significant physical disabilities. She had little use of her left arm and walking with a cane was possible but difficult. She wasn't able to return to work, and although she would have preferred to leave her job on her own terms, she was lucky to be eligible for retirement. She appreciated the wonderful celebration given by her colleagues. Deidre is a doer and likes to get out and about—she has no intention of letting her stroke get in the way of that. It might have slowed down her walking, but she certainly was not going to stop doing the things she enjoyed. When she talked about refusing to cancel a trip to Hawaii with her sons, she said, "I don't know if I can walk on the beach, but we'll figure it out."

MARK WELLS

On July 1, 2013, Mark Wells stepped off a plane excited to be starting a relaxing vacation in Orlando with his new fiancée. He received the worst phone call any father could imagine; back in his hometown of St. Louis, his son had been murdered. He flew home immediately, and four days later Mark suffered a severe stroke. At fifty-eight years old, he had the unthinkable challenge of dealing with substantial physical disabilities while grieving the horrific loss of his son. He says he was never suicidal, but he did share that he often thought he might be better off dead.

Mark, a religious African-American man, largely credits an intensified connection with his faith for his ability to reframe his narrative from one of grief and despair to one of commitment and hope. He learned to trust God and be content with his place in the world, despite the circumstances. He was clear that this has been anything but easy and that, for some time, it was a near daily battle to stay positive. Mark is extremely thankful that he still has all of his cognitive abilities and was able to return to his work as an accountant. When asked about how his stroke affected him, he explained, "I'm not the same person now that I was before my stroke." But after a little thought, he continued, "In fact, I'm a better person because I appreciate life more. What matters to me now is passing on how life is precious to my children and people around me."

Maslow's Hierarchy of Needs

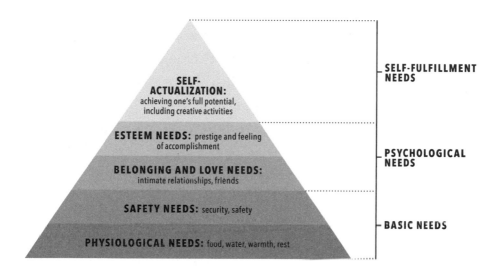

The empirical and theoretical validity of Maslow's hierarchy is hotly debated, but it's certainly a useful tool for thinking about my problem. Maslow's hierarchy gave me a way to understand my desires, frustrations, and challenges—both physical and emotional. There were needs that I could articulate and others that were less obvious, even to me.[135]

BASIC NEEDS: Physiological needs clearly came first. I needed acute medical care. I was completely dependent on others to keep me alive. Since my survival was in doubt, little else mattered. **Safety needs** came next: I was reliant on others for basic security. Like other survivors, I strongly resented my dependence, and this was a cause of massive frustration. Regaining the ability to provide for my own basic needs was an early motivator.

PSYCHOLOGICAL NEEDS: A desire to belong accelerated my poststroke identity crisis. Loss of language was a big issue here, creating gaps within previous relationships and communities. Even once I felt secure and embraced by family and friends, I lacked **self-esteem,** and my previous avenues to build it had closed. I could not teach, ski, or even be a mother as I used to.

SELF-FULFILLMENT NEEDS: As I came to realize that my abilities and options in life were forever changed, the real challenge presented itself. How could I now achieve **self-actualization?** How could I grow as a person when I was now so far removed from the person I had been working on for fifty-three years? My stroke had thrown me off the path I was on, and I had to find a new one.

Notes

INTRODUCTION

1. Debra E. Meyerson, *Tempered Radicals: How People Use Difference to Inspire Change at Work,* (Boston: Harvard Business School Press, 2001). *Rocking the Boat: How Tempered Radicals Effect Change Without Making Trouble* (Boston: Harvard Business School Press, 2008). Citations refer to *Tempered Radicals.*

CHAPTER 1. A SLOW FALL OFF A CLIFF

2. See the Mayo Clinic's website for more: http://www.mayoclinic.org/diseases-conditions/stroke/symptoms-causes/dxc-20117265

3. "Impact of Stroke," American Stroke Association (Accessed May 12, 2015). http://www.strokeassociation.org/STROKEORG/AboutStroke/Impact-of-Stroke-Stroke-statistics_UCM_310728_Article.jsp

4. "The Atlas of Heart Disease and Stroke," World Health Organization (Accessed July 20, 2018). https://www.who.int/cardiovascular_diseases/resources/atlas/en/

5. Kerry Kuluski, Clare Dow, Louise Locock, Renee F. Lyons, and Daniel Lasseron, "Life Interrupted and Life Regained? Coping with Stroke at a Young Age," *International Journal of Qualitative Studies on Health and Well-Being* 23 (January 23, 2014): 1-12.

6. For more signs of stroke, visit the Henry Ford Allegiance Health Center website: https://www.allegiancehealth.org/services/heart-vascular/signs-heart-attack-or-stroke

7. Jill Bolte Taylor, *My Stroke of Insight: A Brain Scientist's Personal Journey* (New York: Penguin Books, 2006).

CHAPTER 2. **EVERYTHING CAN FAIL**

8. Sharon R. Kaufman, "Toward a Phenomenology of Boundaries in Medicine: Chronic Illness Experience in the Case of Stroke," *Medical Anthropology Quarterly* 2, no. 4 (December 1988): 341.

9. Ibid.

10. Lauren Marks, *A Stitch of Time: The Year a Brain Injury Changed My Language and Life* (New York: Simon & Schuster, 2017).

CHAPTER 3. **A TEACHER WITHOUT WORDS**

11. Meyerson, *Tempered Radicals*, xi.

12. Eric H. Erikson, *Identity: Youth and Crisis* (New York: W.W. Norton & Company, 1968).

13. Sharon Anderson and Kyle Whitfield, "Social Identity and Stroke: 'They Don't Make Me Feel Like, There's Something Wrong with Me,'" *Scandinavian Journal of Caring Sciences* 27 (2013): 821.

14. Amara T. Brook, Julie Garcia, and Monique A. Fleming, "The Effects of Multiple Identities on Psychological Well-Being," *Personality and Social Psychology Bulletin* 34, no. 1 (2008): 600.

15. Paul Kalanithi, *When Breath Becomes Air* (New York: Random House, 2016): 38.

16. Kuluski et al., "Life Interrupted and Life Regained? Coping with Stroke at a Young Age": 1-12.

17. Sally Maitlis, "Who Am I Now? Sensemaking and Identity in Posttraumatic Growth," *Exploring Positive Identities and Organizations: Building a Theoretical and Research Foundation*, edited by Laura Morgan Roberts and Jane E. Dutton, (New York: Routledge, 2009): 49.

18. Meyerson, *Tempered Radicals*: 60.

19. Kenneth Gergen, *The Saturated Self: Dilemmas of Identity in Contemporary Life* (New York: Basic Books, 2000): 139.

20. Lakshmi Ramarajan, "Past, Present and Future Research on Multiple Identities: Toward an Intrapersonal Network Approach," *The Academy of Management Annals* 8, no. 1 (2014): 589-659.

21. Peter E. Burke, *Contemporary Social Psychological Theories* (Palo Alto, CA: Stanford University Press, 2006).

22. Abraham H. Maslow, *Theory of Human Motivation* (Jersey City, NJ: Start Publishing, 2012). Abridged from A.H. Maslow, "A Theory of Human Motivation," 50 *Psychological Review* (1943): 370-396.

CHAPTER 4. **MOVING FORWARD**

23. Kuluski et al., "Life Interrupted and Life Regained?": 1-12.

24. Sheryl Sandberg and Adam Grant, *Option B: Facing Adversity, Building Resilience, and Finding Joy* (New York: Knopf, 2017): 174-175.

25. Karl E. Weick, "Small Wins: Redefining the Scale of Social Problems," *American Psychologist* 39, no. 1 (1984): 40-49.

26. Meyerson, *Tempered Radicals*: 101-120.

27. Sandberg and Grant, *Option B*: 23.

28. Philip Brickman and Donald Campbell, "Hedonic Relativism and Planning the Good Society," in *Adaptation Level Theory: A Symposium*, edited by M. II. Apley (New York: Academic Press, 1971): 287-330.

29. Philip Brickman, Dan Coates, and Ronnie Janoff-Bulman. "Lottery Winners and Accident Victims: Is Happiness Relative?" *Journal of Personality and Social Psychology* 36, no. 8 (1978): 917-927.

30. Karl E. Weick, *Sensemaking in Organizations: Foundations for Organizational Science* (Thousand Oaks, CA: Sage Publications, 1995): 18-24.

31. Maitlis, "Who Am I Now?": 48-49.

32. Ibid, 49.

33. Laure L. Wang, *Reflections on a Changed Life* (Taiwan: Pacific Venture Partners, 2015).

34. Jonathan Haidt, *The Righteous Mind: Why Good People Are Divided by Politics and Religion* (New York: Vintage Books, 2013).

35. Sandberg and Grant, *Option B*: 20-23.

CHAPTER 5. **THE GRIND OF THERAPY**

36. Kaufman, "Toward a Phenomenology of Boundaries in Medicine: Chronic Illness Experience in the Case of Stroke": 342.

37. Weick, "Small Wins: Redefining the Scale of Social Problems": 40.

38. Teresa M. Amabile and Steven J. Kramer. "The Power of Small Wins," *Harvard Business Review* (May 2011).

39. Tevicker, "Sean Maloney rowing video," YouTube video (Posted Feb 16, 2011). https://www.youtube.com/watch?v=iiIpOK46LYg&t=2s

40. Kaufman, "Toward a Phenomenology of Boundaries in Medicine: Chronic Illness Experience in the Case of Stroke": 342.

CHAPTER 6. **LET ME TALK!**

41. Dr. Mike Dow and David Dow, *Healing the Broken Brain* (Hay House, Inc., 2017): 70. David Dow, who suffered a stroke when he was ten years old, also wrote along with Dr. Mike Dow and Carol Dow-Richards, *Brain Attack: My Journey of Recovery from Stroke and Aphasia* (Speechless Publishing, 2013).

42. Leora R. Cherney, Janet P. Patterson, and Anastasia M. Raymer, "Intensity of Aphasia Therapy: Evidence and Efficacy," *Current Neurology and Neuroscience Reports* 11, (2011): 560.

43 M.A. LeMay, "The Person with Aphasia and Society," in *Living with Aphasia: Psychosocial Issues*, edited by D. Lafond et al. (Norwich, United Kingdom: Singular, 1993): 212.

44. Oliver Sacks, *The Mind's Eye* (New York: Vintage, 2010): 41.

45. Barbara B. Shadden and Joseph P. Agan, "Renegotiation of Identity: The Social Context of Aphasia Support Groups," *Topics in Language Disorders* 24, no. 3 (September 2004): 174-186.

46. Tom Wolfe, *The Kingdom of Speech* (New York: Little Brown & Company, 2016): 5.

47. Berit Arnesveen et al., "Psychosocial Well-Being in Persons with Aphasia Participating in a Nursing Intervention after Stroke," *Nursing Research and Practice* (2012): 1-14.

48. Barbara B. Shadden, "Aphasia As Identity Theft: Theory and Practice," *Aphasiology* 19 (2005): 216.

49. Ibid.

50. Dr. Albert Mehrabian, author of *Silent Messages*. He found that, on average, 7 percent of any message is conveyed through words, 38 percent through certain vocal elements, and 55 percent through nonverbal elements (facial expressions, gestures, posture, etc.). http://www.nonverbalgroup.com/2011/08/how-much-of-communication-is-really-nonverbal

51. Sacks, *The Mind's Eye:* 41.

CHAPTER 7. **GRIEF**

52. "Depression Trumps Recovery," *StrokeConnection* (September/October 2003).

53. Elisabeth Kübler-Ross, *On Death and Dying* (New York: Scribner, 1969).

54. Jon Caswell and Rachel Scanlon Henry, "Grieving the Old Self, Embracing the New," *StrokeConnection* (Fall 2017).

55. Kathy Charmaz, "Loss of Self: A Fundamental Form of Suffering in the Chronically Ill," *Sociology of Health and Illness* 5, no. 2 (1983).

56. Jonathan Haidt, *The Happiness Hypothesis: Finding Modern Truth in Ancient Wisdom* (New York: Basic Books, 2006).

57. Jon Caswell, "Helping Others Understand: Post-Stroke Depression," *StrokeConnection* (Spring 2008).

58. Sandberg and Grant, *Option B*: 13.

CHAPTER 8. **LEAN ON**

59. Heather R. Walen and Margie E. Lachman, "Social Support and Strain from Partner, Family, and Friends: Costs and Benefits for Men and Women in Adulthood," *Journal of Social and Personal Relationships* 17, no. 1 (2000): 6.

60. Jenni Murray, John Young, Anne Forster, and Robert Ashworth, "Developing a Primary Care-Based Stroke Model: The Prevalence of Longer-Term Problems Experienced by Patients and Carers," *British Journal of General Practice* 53 (2003): 803-807.

61. Sandberg and Grant, *Option B*: 39.

62. Anderson and Whitfield, "Social Identity and Stroke: 'They Don't Make Me Feel Like, There's Something Wrong with Me'": 821.

63. Sandberg and Grant, *Option B*: 52.

CHAPTER 9. **STROKE IS A FAMILY ILLNESS**

64. Gabriele Kitzmüller, Kenneth Asplund, and Terttu Häggström, "The Long-Term Experience of Family Life After Stroke," *Journal of Neuroscience Nursing* 44, no. 1 (February 2012): E3.

65. Ibid, E4.

CHAPTER 10. **PARTNERS AND INTIMACY**

66. Ibid, E6.

67. Bella DePaulo, "What Is the Divorce Rate, Really? Is It True that Half of All Marriages End in Divorce?" *Psychology Today* (February 2, 2017).

68. Kitzmüller et al., "The Long-Term Experience of Family Life After Stroke": E7.

69. Ibid.

70. Trish Reay, Karen Golden-Biddle, and Kathy Germann, "Legitimizing a New Role: Small Wins and Microprocesses of Change," *Academy of Management Journal* 49, no. 5 (2006): 990.

71. Jon Caswell, "Sex and Intimacy after Stroke," *StrokeConnection* (March-April 2009).

72. Reg Morris, "The Psychology of Stroke in Young Stroke Adults: The Role of Service Provision and Return to Work," *Stroke Research and Treatment* (March 2011). https://www.ncbi.nlm.nih.gov/pmc/articles/PMC3056452/

73. Caswell, "Sex and Intimacy after Stroke."

74. Meghann Jane Grawburg, "Investigating Third-Party Functioning and Third-Party Disability in Family Members of People with Aphasia." Dissertation, University of Canterbury, New Zealand (October 2013).

75. Kitzmüller et al., "The Long-Term Experience of Family Life After Stroke": E4.

CHAPTER 11. **PEOPLE ARE SOCIAL ANIMALS**

76. David Brooks, *The Road to Character* (New York: Random House, 2015).

77. Gergen, *The Saturated Self.*

78. Kitzmüller et al., "The Long-Term Experience of Family Life After Stroke."

79. Jennifer Guise, Andy McKinlay, and Sue Widdicombe, "The Impact of Early Stroke on Identity: A Discourse Analytic Study," *Health* 14, no. 1 (2010): 76.

80. Guise et al., "The Impact of Early Stroke on Identity: A Discourse Analytic Study": 79.

81. Anderson and Whitfield, "Social Identity and Stroke": 820.

82. Ibid.

83. Ramarajan, "Past, Present and Future Research on Multiple Identities": 589-659.

84. Maitlis, "Who Am I Now?": 50.

CHAPTER 12. **HOW THE WORLD RESPONDS**

85. United States Census (July 25, 2012). https://www.census.gov/newsroom/releases/archives/miscellaneous/cb12-134.html

86. Meyerson, *Tempered Radicals*: 39-42.

87. Christopher A. Faircloth et al., "Sudden Illness and Biographical Flow in Narratives of Stroke Recovery," *Sociology of Health and Illness*. 26, no. 2 (March 2004): 242-261.

88. Maitlis, "Who Am I Now?": 68. "Master status" was Robert Merton, 1957.

89. Faircloth et al., "Sudden Illness and Biographical Flow in Narratives of Stroke Recovery": 243.

90. Faircloth et al., "Sudden Illness and Biographical Flow: 248-249."

91. Meyerson, *Tempered Radicals*: 42.

CHAPTER 13. **ACTIVITIES ADAPTED**

92. Mihály Csíkszentmihályi, *Flow: The Psychology of Optimal Experience* (New York: HarperCollins, 1991).

93. Maitlis, "Who Am I Now?": 50.

94. Ibid.

CHAPTER 14. **CAREERS AND CALLINGS**

95. Mike G. Pratt and Blake E. Ashforth, "Fostering Meaningfulness in Working and at Work," *Positive Organizational Scholarship,* edited by Kim S. Cameron, Jane E. Dutton, and Robert E. Quinn (San Francisco, Berrett-Koehler Publishers, 2003): 307.

96. Kuluski et al. "Life Interrupted and Life Regained?": 222-252.

97. Barbara Wolfenden and Marty Grace, "Vulnerability and Post-Stroke Experiences of Working-Age Survivors During Recovery," Sage Publishing Open Access (October-December, 2015): 1-14.

98. Benjamin Musser, Joanne Wilkinson, Thomas Gilbert, and Barbara G. Bokhour, "Changes in Identity after Aphasic Stroke: Implications for Primary Care," *International Journal of Family Medicine* (2015): 3.

99. John P. Robinson and Geoffrey Godbey, *Time for Life: The Surprising Ways Americans Use Their Time,* foreword by Robert D. Putnam, xvi (University Park, Pennsylvania: The Pennsylvania State University Press, 1997).

100. Wolfenden and Grace, "Identity Continuity in the Face of Biographical Disruption: 'It's the same me.'" *Brain Impairment* 13, no. 2 (September 2012): 206.

101. Musser et al., "Changes in Identity after Aphasic Stroke": 4.

102. Maitlis, "Who Am I Now?": 68.

103. Weick, "Small Wins": 40.

104. Maitlis, "Who Am I Now?": 68.

105. Ibid.

106. Justin M. Berg, Adam M. Grant, and Victoria Johnson, "When Callings Are Calling: Crafting Work and Leisure in Pursuit of Unanswered Occupational Callings," *Organization Science* 21, no. 5 (September-October 2010): 973-994.

107. Julia Fox Garrison, *Don't Leave Me This Way: Or When I Get Back on My Feet You'll Be Sorry* (New York: Harper Collins, 2006).

108. Amy Wrzesniewski, Kathryn H. Dekas, and Brent Rosso, "Callings," In S. Lopez & A. Beauchamp (Eds.), *Encyclopedia of Positive Psychology* (Oxford, United Kingdom: Blackwell, 2009).

CHAPTER 15. **DEALING WITH FINANCIAL STRAIN**

109. *Finances After Stroke Guide*, American Heart Association/American Stroke Association (2014). http://www.strokeassociation.org/idc/groups/stroke-public/@ wcm/@hcm/@sta/documents/downloadable/ucm_489492.pdf

110. Tami Luhby, "America's Middle Class: Poorer than You Think," CNN (August 5, 2014).

111. "Health Insurance Coverage in the United States: 2016," United State Census (September 2017).

112. Joel N. Swerdel et al., "Ischemic Stroke Rate Increases in Young Adults: Evidence for a Generational Effect?," *Journal of the American Heart Association* (2016). https://www.ahajournals.org/doi/abs/10.1161/jaha.116.004245

113. Mary G. George, Xin Tong, and Barbara A. Bowman, "Prevalence of Cardiovascular Risk Factors and Strokes in Younger Adults," *JAMA Neurology* (June 2017).

114. Inequality.org (October 2018). https://inequality.org/

CHAPTER 16. **ADVOCATING IN THE U.S. MEDICAL SYSTEM**

115. Charmaz, "Loss of Self: A Fundamental Form of Suffering in the Chronically Ill": 169.

116. Julia Fox Garrison, *Don't Leave Me This Way* (New York: HarperCollins, 2006).

CHAPTER 17. **RECLAIMING THE BASICS**

117. Atul Gawande, *Being Mortal: Illness, Medicine and What Matters in the End* (New York: Metropolitan Books, 2014): 243.

118. Kaufman, "Toward a Phenomenology of Boundaries in Medicine": 347.

119. Faircloth et al., "Sudden Illness and Biographical Flow": 256.

120. Weick, "Small Wins": 43.

121. Kaufman, "Toward a Phenomenology of Boundaries in Medicine": 349.

122. Ibid.

CHAPTER 18. **CHOICE IN OUR NEW IDENTITIES**

123. Robert McCrum, "Deficits," chapter in *My Year Off: Recovering Life After a Stroke* (New York: Broadway Books, 1999).

124. Maitlis, "Who Am I Now?": 48.

125. Caroline S. Ellis-Hill and Sandra Horn, "Change in Identity and Self-Concept: A New Theoretical Approach to Recovery Following Stroke," *Clinical Rehabilitation* 14 (2000): 280.

126. Maitlis, "Who Am I Now?": 50.

127. Jim Rohn, 7 *Strategies for Wealth & Happiness: Power Ideas from America's Foremost Business Philosopher* (New York: Three Rivers Press, 1996).

128. Barbara Shadden, "Aphasia As Identity Theft: Theory and Practice," *Aphasiology,* 19 (2005): 215.

129. Charles H. Vogl, *The Art of Community: Seven Principles for Belonging* (Oakland, CA: Berrett-Koehler Publishers, 2016).

130. Weick, "Small Wins:" 44.

131. Kathy Charmaz, "A Constructivist Grounded Theory Analysis of Losing and Regaining a Valued Self," chapter in Frederick J. Wertz, Kathy Charmaz, Linda J. McMullen, Ruthellen Josselson, Rosemarie Anderson, and Emalinda McSpadden's *Five Ways of Doing Qualitative Analysis: Phenomenological Psychology, Grounded Theory, Discourse Analysis, Narrative Research, and Intuitive Inquiry* (New York: Guilford, 2011): 182.

132. Charmaz, "A Constructivist Grounded Theory Analysis of Losing and Regaining a Valued Self": 179.

CHAPTER 19. **FULFILLMENT THROUGH GROWTH**

133. Csíkszentmihályi, *Flow.* https://positivepsychologyprogram.com/mihaly-csikszentmihalyi-father-of-flow/

134. Victor E. Frankl, *Man's Search for Meaning* (Boston: Beacon Press, 1959).

APPENDIX II. **MASLOW'S HIERARCHY OF NEEDS**

135. Abraham H. Maslow, *Theory of Human Motivation* (Jersey City, NJ: Start Publishing, 2012). Abridged from A.H. Maslow, "A Theory of Human Motivation," 50 *Psychological Review* (1943): 370-396.

References

Amabile, Teresa M. and Steven J. Kramer. "The Power of Small Wins." *Harvard Business Review* (May 2011).

American Heart Association. *Finances After Stroke Guide* (2014). http://www.strokeassociation.org/idc/groups/stroke-public/@wcm/@hcm/@sta/documents/downloadable/ucm_489492.pdf

American Stroke Association. "Impact of Stroke" (Accessed May 12, 2015). http://www.strokeassociation.org/STROKEORG/AboutStroke/Impact-of-Stroke-Stroke-statistics_UCM_310728_Article.jsp

Anderson, Sharon and Kyle Whitfield. "Social Identity and Stroke: 'They Don't Make Me Feel Like, There's Something Wrong with Me.'" *Scandinavian Journal of Caring Sciences* 27 (2013): 820-830.

Arnesveen, Berit et al. "Psychosocial Well-Being in Persons with Aphasia Participating in a Nursing Intervention after Stroke." *Nursing Research and Practice* (2012): 1-14.

Berg, Justin M., Adam M. Grant, and Victoria Johnson. "When Callings Are Calling: Crafting Work and Leisure in Pursuit of Unanswered Occupational Calling." *Organization Science* 21, no. 5 (September-October 2010): 973-994.

Bolte Taylor, Jill. *My Stroke of Insight: A Brain Scientist's Personal Journey* (New York: Penguin Books, 2006).

Brickman, Philip, Dan Coates, and Ronnie Janoff-Bulman. "Lottery Winners and Accident Victims: Is Happiness Relative?" *Journal of Personality and Social Psychology* 36, no. 8 (1978): 917-927.

Brickman, Philip and Donald Campbell. "Hedonic Relativism and Planning the Good Society." In *Adaptation Level Theory: A Symposium*, edited by M. H. Apley (New York: Academic Press, 1971): 287-330.

Brook, Amara T., Julie Garcia, and Monique A. Fleming. "The Effects of Multiple Identities on Psychological Well-Being." *Personality and Social Psychology Bulletin* 34, no. 1 (2008): 1,588-1,600.

Brooks, David. *The Road to Character* (New York: Random House, 2015).

Burke, Peter J. *Contemporary Social Psychological Theories* (Palo Alto, CA: Stanford University Press, 2006).

Caswell, Jon. "Helping Others Understand: Post-Stroke Depression." *StrokeConnection* (Spring 2008).

Caswell, Jon. "Sex and Intimacy after Stroke." *StrokeConnection* (March–April 2009). http://strokeconnection.strokeassociation.org/Mar-Apr-2009/Sex-and-Intimacy-after-Stroke/

Caswell, Jon and Rachel Scanlon Henry. "Grieving the Old Self, Embracing the New." *StrokeConnection* (Fall 2017).

Charmaz, Kathy. "A Constructivist Grounded Theory Analysis of Losing and Regaining a Valued Self" chapter in *Five Ways of Doing Qualitative Analysis: Phenomenological Psychology, Grounded Theory, Discourse Analysis, Narrative Research, and Intuitive Inquiry,* by Frederick J. Wertz, Kathy Charmaz, Linda M. McMullen, Ruthellen Josselson, Rosemarie Anderson, and Emalinda McSpadden (New York: Guilford, 2011: 165-204).

Charmaz, Kathy. "Loss of Self: A Fundamental Form of Suffering in the Chronically Ill." *Sociology of Health & Illness* 5, no. 2 (1983).

Cherney, Leora R., Janet P. Patterson, and Anastasia M. Raymer. "Intensity of Aphasia Therapy: Evidence and Efficacy." *Current Neurology and Neuroscience Reports* 11 (2011): 560-569.

Csíkszentmihályi, Mihály. *Flow: The Psychology of Optimal Experience* (New York: HarperCollins, 1991).

DePaulo, Bella. "What Is the Divorce Rate, Really? Is It True that Half of All Marriages End in Divorce?" *Psychology Today* (Feb. 2, 2017). https://www.psychologytoday.com/us/blog/living-single/201702/what-is-the-divorce-rate-really

"Depression Trumps Recovery." *StrokeConnection* (September/October 2003).

Dow, Mike and David Dow. *Healing the Broken Brain* (Hay House, Inc., 2017).

Ellis-Hill, Caroline S. and Sandra Horn. "Change in Identity and Self-Concept: A New Theoretical Approach to Recovery Following a Stroke." *Clinical Rehabilitation* 14 (2000): 279-287.

Erikson, Eric H. *Identity: Youth and Crisis.* (New York: W.W. Norton & Company, 1968).

Faircloth, Christopher A. et al. "Sudden Illness and Biographical Flow in Narratives of Stroke Recovery." *Sociology of Health and Illness* 26, no. 2 (March 2004).

Fox Garrison, Julia. *Don't Leave Me This Way: Or When I Get Back on My Feet You'll Be Sorry* (New York: Harper Collins, 2006).

Frankl, Victor E. *Man's Search for Meaning* (Boston: Beacon Press, 1959).

Gawande, Atul. *Being Mortal: Illness, Medicine and What Matters in the End* (New York: Metropolitan Books, 2014).

George, Mary G., Xin Tong, and Barbara A. Bowman. "Prevalence of Cardiovascular Risk Factors and Strokes in Younger Adults." *JAMA Neurology* (June 2017).

Gergen, Kenneth J. *The Saturated Self: Dilemmas of Identity in Contemporary Life* (New York: Basic Books, 2000).

Grawburg, Meghann Jane. "Investigating Third-Party Functioning and Third-Party Disability in Family Members of People with Aphasia." Dissertation, University of Canterbury, New Zealand (October 2013).

Guise, Jennifer, Andy McKinlay, and Sue Widdicombe. "The Impact of Early Stroke on Identity: A Discourse Analytic Study." *Health* 14, no. 1 (2010): 75-90.

Haidt, Jonathan. *The Happiness Hypothesis: Finding Modern Truth in Ancient Wisdom* (New York: Basic Books, 2006).

Haidt, Jonathan. *The Righteous Mind: Why Good People Are Divided by Politics and Religion* (New York: Vintage Books, 2013).

Henry Ford Allegiance Health Center website: https://www.allegiancehealth.org/services/heart-vascular/signs-heart-attack-or-stroke

Inequality.org (Accessed October 2018). https://inequality.org/

Kalanithi, Paul. *When Breath Becomes Air* (New York: Random House, 2016).

Kaufman, Sharon R. "Toward a Phenomenology of Boundaries in Medicine: Chronic Illness Experience in the Case of Stroke." *Medical Anthropology Quarterly* 2, no. 4 (December 1988): 338-354.

Kitzmüller, Gabriele, Kenneth Asplund, and Terttu Häggström. "The Long-Term Experience of Family Life After Stroke." *Journal of Neuroscience Nursing* 44, no. 1 (February 2012).

Kübler-Ross, Elisabeth. *On Death and Dying* (New York: Scribner, 1969).

Kuluski, Kerry, Clare Dow, Louise Locock, Renee F. Lyons, and Daniel Lasseron. "Life Interrupted and Life Regained? Coping with Stroke at a Young Age." *International Journal of Qualitative Studies on Health and Well-Being* (January 23, 2014): 1-12.

LeMay, M.A. "The Person with Aphasia and Society." In *Living with Aphasia: Psychosocial Issues*, edited by D. Lafond et al. (Norwich, United Kingdom: Singular, 1993).

Luhby, Tami. "America's Middle Class: Poorer than You Think." CNN (August 5, 2014).

Maitlis, Sally. "Who Am I Now? Sensemaking and Identity in Posttraumatic Growth." *Exploring Positive Identities and Organizations: Building a Theoretical and Research Foundation*, edited by Laura Morgan Roberts and Jane E. Dutton (New York: Routledge, 2009): 47-76.

Marks, Lauren. *A Stitch of Time: The Year a Brain Injury Changed My Language and Life* (New York: Simon & Schuster, 2017).

Maslow, Abraham H. *Theory of Human Motivation* (Jersey City, NJ: Start Publishing, 2012). Abridged from A.H. Maslow, "A Theory of Human Motivation," *Psychological Review* 50 (1943): 370-396.

Mayo Clinic. "Stroke." http://www.mayoclinic.org/diseases-conditions/stroke/symptoms-causes/dxc-20117265

McCrum, Robert. *My Year Off: Recovering Life After a Stroke* (New York: Broadway Books, 1999).

Meyerson, Debra E. *Tempered Radicals: How People Use Difference to Inspire Change at Work* (Boston: Harvard Business School Press, 2001). *Rocking the Boat: How Tempered Radicals Effect Change Without Making Trouble* (Boston: Harvard Business School Press, 2008). Citations refer to *Tempered Radicals*.

Morris, Reg. "The Psychology of Stroke in Young Stroke Adults: The Role of Service Provision and Return to Work." *Stroke Research and Treatment* (March 2011). https://www.ncbi.nlm.nih.gov/pmc/articles/PMC3056452/

Murray, Jenni, John Young, Anne Forster, and Robert Ashworth. "Developing a Primary Care-Based Stroke Model: The Prevalence of Longer-Term Problems Experienced by Patients and Carers." *British Journal of General Practice* 53 (2003): 803-807.

Musser, Benjamin, Joanne Wilkinson, Thomas Gilbert, and Barbara G. Bokhour. "Changes in Identity After Aphasic Stroke: Implications for Primary Care." *International Journal of Family Medicine* (2015).

Pratt, Mike G. and Blake E. Ashforth. "Fostering Meaningfulness in Working and at Work." *Positive Organizational Scholarship*, edited by Kim S. Cameron, Jane E. Dutton, and Robert E. Quinn. (San Francisco: Berrett-Koehler Publishers, 2003): 307-327.

Ramarajan, Lakshmi. "Past, Present and Future Research on Multiple Identities: Toward an Intrapersonal Network Approach." *The Academy of Management Annals* 8, no. 1 (2014): 589-659.

Reay, Trish, Karen Golden-Biddle, and Kathy Germann. "Legitimizing a New Role: Small Wins and Microprocesses of Change." *Academy of Management Journal* 49, no. 5 (2006): 977-998.

Robinson, John P. and Geoffrey Godbey. *Time for Life: The Surprising Ways Americans Use Their Time.* Foreword by Robert D. Putnam, xvi (University Park, Pennsylvania: The Pennsylvania State University Press, 1997).

Rohn, Jim. *7 Strategies for Wealth & Happiness: Power Ideas from America's Foremost Business Philosopher* (New York: Three Rivers Press, 1996).

Sacks, Oliver. *The Mind's Eye* (New York: Vintage, 2010).

Sandberg, Sheryl and Adam Grant. *Option B: Facing Adversity, Building Resilience, and Finding Joy.* (New York: Knopf, 2017).

Shadden, Barbara B. "Aphasia As Identity Theft: Theory and Practice." *Aphasiology* 19 (2005): 211-223.

Shadden, Barbara B. and Joseph P. Agan. "Renegotiation of Identity: The Social Context of Aphasia Support Groups." *Topics in Language Disorders* 24, no. 3 (September 2004): 174-186.

Swerdel, Joel N. et al. "Ischemic Stroke Rate Increases in Young Adults: Evidence for a Generational Effect?" *Journal of the American Heart Association* (2016). https://www.ahajournals.org/doi/abs/10.1161/jaha.116.004245

Tevicker, YouTube. "Sean Maloney rowing video" (Posted February 16, 2011). https://www.youtube.com/watch?v=iiIpOK46LYg&t=2s

United States Census. "Health Insurance Coverage in the United States: 2016," (September 2017).

United States Census. "Nearly 1 in 5 People Have a Disability in the U.S., Census Bureau Reports," (July 25, 2012). https://www.census.gov/newsroom/releases/archives/miscellaneous/cb12-134.html

Vogl, Charles H. *The Art of Community: Seven Principles for Belonging* (Oakland, CA: Berrett-Koehler Publishers, 2016).

Walen, Heather R. and Margie E. Lachman. "Social Support and Strain from Partner, Family, and Friends: Costs and Benefits for Men and Women in Adulthood." *Journal of Social and Personal Relationships* 17, no. 1 (2000): 5-30.

Wang, Laure L. *Reflections on a Changed Life* (Taiwan: Pacific Venture Partners, 2015).

Weick, Karl E. *Sensemaking in Organizations: Foundations for Organizational Science* (Thousand Oaks, CA: Sage Publications, 1995): 18-24.

Weick, Karl E. "Small Wins: Redefining the Scale of Social Problems." *American Psychologist* 39, no. 1 (1984): 40-49.

Wolfe, Tom. *The Kingdom of Speech* (New York: Little Brown & Company, 2016).

Wolfenden, Barbara and Marty Grace. "Identity Continuity in the Face of Biographical Disruption: 'It's the Same Me.'" *Brain Impairment* 13, no. 2 (Sept 2012): 203-211.

Wolfenden, Barbara and Marty Grace. "Vulnerability and Post-Stroke Experiences of Working-Age Survivors During Recovery." Sage Publishing Open Access (October-December, 2015): 1-14.

World Health Organization. Cerebrovascular Disorders: "The Atlas of Heart Disease and Stroke." (July 20, 2018). https://www.who.int/cardiovascular_diseases/resources/atlas/en/

Wrzesniewski, Amy, Kathryn H. Dekas and Brent Rosso. "Callings" in *Encyclopedia of Positive Psychology*, edited by S. Lopez and A. Beauchamp (Oxford, United Kingdom: Blackwell, 2009).

Index

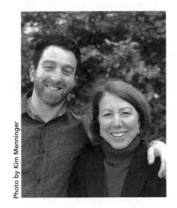

Photo by Kim Menninger

About the Authors

Previously a tenured professor at Stanford University, Debra Meyerson studied, wrote, lectured, and taught about diversity, gender, identity, and organizational change. In September 2010, Debra's life and career were derailed by a severe stroke that nearly killed her and initially left her paralyzed on the right side—and completely mute. Years of intensive therapy and a relentless work ethic enabled Debra to regain her independence, but she still lives with physical limitations and speech challenges. Debra wrote *Identity Theft* to help other survivors and those closest to them navigate the emotional journey that she has found very difficult—and rewarding. Debra lives in Menlo Park, California, with her husband, and has three grown children.

Danny Zuckerman is the cofounder of 3Box, a peer-to-peer social network that helps people create more meaningful connections and communities online. He previously worked on a new digital identity system based on blockchain technology, helped build digital math curriculum at Zearn, worked as a management consultant at Bain & Company, and studied political philosophy and economics at Stanford University. Danny is Debra Meyerson's son.

Andrews McMeel Publishing
a division of Andrews McMeel Universal
1130 Walnut Street, Kansas City, Missouri 64106

www.andrewsmcmeel.com

www.identitytheftbook.org
www.stroke-forward.org
www.debmeyerson.com

19 20 21 22 23 BVG 10 9 8 7 6 5 4 3 2 1

ISBN paperback: 978-1-4494-9630-2
ISBN hardcover: 978-1-4494-9631-9

Library of Congress Control Number: 2018966588

Editor: Jean Z. Lucas
Art Director/Designer: Diane Marsh
Production Editor: Elizabeth A. Garcia
Production Manager: Carol Coe

Illustration © rosendo/Getty Images